18 NATURAL WAYS
TO STOP
ARTHRITIS
NOW

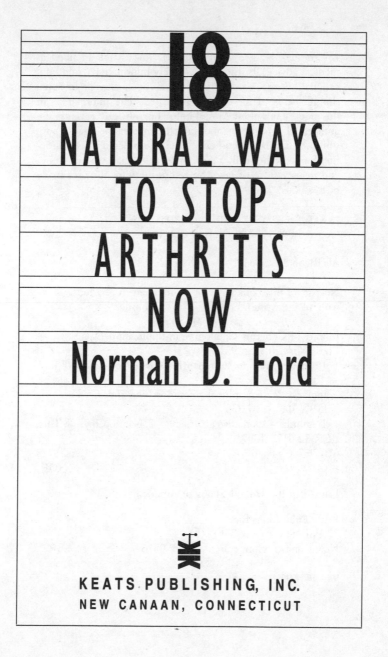

18
NATURAL WAYS
TO STOP
ARTHRITIS
NOW
Norman D. Ford

KEATS PUBLISHING, INC.
NEW CANAAN, CONNECTICUT

18 Natural Ways to Stop Arthritis Now is not intended as medical advice. Its intention is solely informational and educational. Please consult a medical or health professional should the need for one be indicated. The information in this book lends itself to self-help. For obvious reasons, the author and publisher cannot take the medical or legal responsibility of having the contents herein considered as a prescription for everyone. Either you, or the physician who examines and treats you, must take the resonsibility for the uses made of this book.

18 NATURAL WAYS TO STOP ARTHRITIS NOW
Copyright © 1997 by Norman D. Ford

Library of Congress Cataloging-in-Publication Data
Ford, Norman D., 1921–
  18 natural ways to stop arthritis now / Norman D. Ford.
    p. cm.
  Includes bibliographical references and index.
  ISBN 0-87983-726-8
  1. Arthritis—Alternative treatment. 2. Naturopathy. I. Title.
RC933.F645 1997
616.7'2206—dc20   96-35723
                                                            CIP

Printed in the United States of America

Keats Publishing, Inc.
27 Pine Street (Box 876)
New Canaan, Connecticut 06840-0876

98 97 96   6 5 4 3 2 1

ACKNOWLEDGMENTS

Few of the ideas in this book are actually mine. As a health reporter, my role in writing this book was to search out the best discoveries and findings of America's leading researchers and practitioners of nondrug treatments for arthritis. I then organized them into a single self-care program that anyone could use. In the process, I drew on hundreds of documented studies authored by prominent researchers in the fields of arthritis, immunology, behavioral medicine and related sciences. Regrettably, it is impossible to acknowledge them all.

However, I must acknowledge my debt to the extensive research carried out by the Arthritis Foundation of Atlanta; and by Herbert Benson, M.D., Mindbody Medical Institute, Harvard Medical School; John H. Bland, M.D., Professor of Medicine, University of Vermont College of Medicine; John Bogden, Ph.D., Professor of Preventive Medicine and Community Health,, New Jersey Medical School, Newark, N.J.; Joan Borysenko, Ph.D., Mindbody Health Sciences Inc.; Robert S. Elliot, M.D., Institute of Stress Medicine; William J. Evans, Ph.D., Director, Physiological Research Center, Pennsylvania State University; Gregory Heath, D.H.Sc., Exercise Physiologist, Center for Disease Control, Atlanta; Joel

M. Kremer, M.D., Division of Rheumatology, Albany Medical College, N.Y.; Dean M. Ornish, M.D., Preventive Medicine Research Institute, Sausalito, Calif.; Kenneth R. Pelletier, Ph.D., Stanford University, Calif.; James M. Rippe, M.D., Director, University of Massachusetts Exercise Physiology Lab; Bernie S. Siegel, M.D., Woodbridge Conn.; Stephanie Simonton, Ph.D., Behavioral Medicine Program, University of Arkansas; and Lydia Temoshek, Ph.D., World Health Organization, Geneva, Switzerland.

I also drew extensively on research or studies carried out by the Center for Spine, Sports and Rehabilitation, Rehabilitation Institute of Chicago; Framingham Cardiovascular Institute, Framingham, Mass.; National Institute for the Clinical Application of Behavioral Medicine, Mansfield Center, Conn.; National Institute of Allergy and Infectious Diseases, National Institute of Arthritis and Musculoskeletal and Skin Diseases, National Institute of Mental Health, all at Bethesda, Md.; Pacific Northwest Clinical Research Center, Portland, Ore.; Society of Behavioral Medicine, Rockville, Md.; and the Texas Back Institute, Houston, Tex.

I also drew on files and literature from the various multipurpose arthritis centers at major hospitals and university medical centers including: American Institute of Stress, the Mindbody Medical Institute of New England, and the Center for Study of Nutritional Medicine, all at Deaconness Hospital, Boston; Arthritis Center, Brigham and Women's Hospital, Boston; Boston University Arthritis Center; Division of Rheumatic Diseases, University of Connecticut Health Center, Farmington Conn.; Division of Rheumatic Diseases, University of Texas Southwest Medical Center, Dallas, Tex.; Duke University Arthritis Center, Durham, N.C.; Immunochemistry Lab, George Washington University Medical Center, Washington, D.C.; Indiana University

Multipurpose Arthritis & Musculoskeletal Center, Indianapolis; Johns Hopkins Hospital, Baltimore; Mayo Clinic, Rochester, Minn.; Northeast Ohio Multipurpose Arthritis Center, Case Western Reserve University Medical School, Cleveland; Rheumatic Disease Clinic, Cornell University, Ithaca, N.Y.; Section of Rheumatology, Rush-Presbyterian St. Luke's Medical Center, Chicago; Stanford Immunology & Rheumatology Clinic, Stanford University, Stanford, Calif.; Thurston Arthritis Research Center, University of North Carolina, Chapel Hill, N.C.; UAB Arthritis Center, University of Alabama Medical Center, Birmingham, Ala.; and the University of Colorado Center for Human Nutrition, Denver.

Abbreviations Used in This Book

AF	Arthritis Fighter
BMI	Body Mass Index
DMARDs	Disease-Modifying Anti-Rheumatic Drugs
EFA	Essential Fatty Acid
ERT	Estrogen Replacement Therapy
FDA	Food and Drug Administration
HNRC	Jean Mayer Health & Nutrition Research Center on Aging at Tufts University
IU	International Unit(s)
mcg	Micrograms
mg	Milligrams
NSAIDs	Nonsteroid Anti-Inflammatory Drugs
OA	Osteoarthritis
RA	Rheumatoid Arthritis
RDA	Recommended Dietary Allowance
USDA	United States Department of Agriculture

CONTENTS

18 NATURAL WAYS TO STOP ARTHRITIS NOW

CHAPTER ONE

Knock Out Arthritis the Natural Way

You can sit in a uranium mine, take 18 aspirin a day, wear a copper bracelet or take a variety of powerful, chemically active drugs, but you cannot cure arthritis. There is, in fact, no cure for arthritis. But you don't have to go on suffering.

In every area of healing, from drugs to natural alternative therapies, researchers have found effective treatments that can help relieve arthritis pain and symptoms and, in some cases, achieve long periods of total remission.

Yes, drugs are often quite effective in relieving pain and inflammation or in subduing the arthritis process. For many people, though, the adverse side effects of certain drugs are as bad, or even worse, than the pain and discomfort of arthritis itself.

1

Nor are most arthritis drugs a panacea. Despite an avalanche of new and expensive painkillers to hit the market in recent years, low-cost aspirin still remains the most effective drug for pain relief.

Don't Overestimate the Power of Drugs

To battle some forms of arthritis, doctors may prescribe powerful gold salts and antimalarial and immunosuppressive drugs that increase your risk of getting cancer or infections. Drugs like these each have a list of unpleasant side effects so depressingly long that patients have to be constantly monitored by their physician while taking them. As a result, patient compliance is poor and some people stop taking their medication altogether.

When it comes to preventing arthritis pain and incapacity, scores of studies have proven that regular exercise does a far better job of relieving pain and stiffness than any drug or medical treatment. A combination of gentle flexibility exercises combined with a rhythmic exercise like swimming, walking or cycling allows most people with arthritis to function almost normally.

Backlash Against Harsh and Powerful Arthritis Drugs

Widespread concern about the disturbing side effects and low efficacy of many anti-arthritis drugs has promoted a renaissance for natural, nondrug therapies like exercise to beat arthritis.

The purpose of this book is to place at your disposal the 18 best and safest nondrug techniques that have shown real promise in relieving arthritis pain and symptoms. Each of these techniques requires you to use your mind or muscles to perform a physical or mental action-step. In this book, each of these therapeutic action-steps is called an Arthritis Fighter (or AF for short).

Some of our Arthritis Fighters function on the physical level, strengthening muscles that cushion joints and increasing the flexibility of stiff elbows, knees, spine and hips. Others work on the psychological level, calming the mind and reducing stress. Still others work on the nutritional level, providing us with nutrients that help reduce the pain and symptoms of arthritis.

But in addition, each Arthritis Fighter also has a hidden benefit. Whenever we use an AF, it can help to activate tremendous inner healing powers within the body-mind. And a number of scientists working on the cutting edge of arthritis research have suggested that the body's own healing powers may actually have greater capability to conquer arthritis than anything else. This rationale is based on the recent discovery that, in most cases, arthritis is a physical disease that is psychological in origin.

So What Exactly Is Arthritis?

Arthritis is not a single disease. It is an umbrella term for almost 100 different rheumatic diseases, syndromes and conditions that affect the joints or the supportive tissue surrounding them.

Nonarticular rheumatic diseases such as bursitis, fibrositis, tendinitis, or lower back pain are usually mild dysfunctions that affect only soft tissue like muscles, tendons, bursae or ligaments.

Articular rheumatic diseases affect one or more joints and are the really painful, chronic forms of arthritis.

This book deals with the two principal types of articular

3

rheumatic disease: *rheumatoid arthritis* (RA), which affects about 7 million Americans and *osteoarthritis* (OA), which affects about 16 million. Gout, which affects another 2 million Americans (most commonly overweight, sedentary men who indulge in rich foods and alcohol), is also an arthritic disease.

Most people who complain of arthritis have either RA or OA. In both diseases the underlying cause is unresolved emotional stress, and both strike in the joints. But in every other way they are completely different diseases.

RHEUMATOID ARTHRITIS

Rheumatoid arthritis is a progressive, systematic disease that affects the entire body. It most frequently strikes after a period of severe and prolonged stress such as an angry divorce or loss of a spouse or job. Three-fourths of all cases occur in women, particularly between the ages of 35 and 50, the stressful child-raising years. It may also occur in men, usually in later life.

Negative emotions triggered by stress are communicated to the immune system which protects the body against cancer and infectious diseases. In people genetically prone to RA, such stress creates an abnormality in the immune system known as autoimmunity. Autoimmunity is the first stage in the RA process.

The second stage is a series of autoimmune reactions. Right off, autoimmunity causes our immune system to malfunction. Instead of defending the body as it's supposed to, the immune system begins to attack certain cells in our joints. Other autoimmune reactions cause swelling, inflammation and heat in these same afflicted joints. Still other autoimmune reactions may cause poor digestion, low-grade

4

fever, food allergies, fatigue, muscular stiffness and loss of weight and appetite.

In one case in six, RA is severe enough to cause grotesquely distorted joints which may eventually become rigid and fused. While most cases are less severe, the disease progresses in a series of flare-ups and remissions that may be frequent or that may occur months apart. Each year, approximately one person in ten with RA achieves a spontaneous remission which can last for months or years. Or the disease may never return.

Other, less common forms of arthritis which involve the immune system include scleroderma, systematic lupus erythematosus, which primarily affect women, and ankylosing spondylitis, which occurs mainly in men aged 16 to 35. Most Arthritis Fighters which help people with RA are also beneficial for people with these other forms of arthritis but should be used only with a doctor's permission. Arthritis Fighters #15 through #18, which reduce stress, can almost certainly benefit these types of arthritis (as well as fibrositis, a nonarticular rheumatic disease).

OSTEOARTHRITIS

Osteoarthritis is a nonsystematic disease that causes breakdown of bone and cartilage in joints, resulting in restricted mobility. Pain and stiffness are the primary symptoms in the afflicted joints. OA develops slowly, but eventually it wears away cartilage in weight-bearing joints such as the knees, hips and spinal vertebrae; it may also affect shoulders, elbows, wrists and joints in the fingers. Over 16 million Americans have some degree of OA and the majority are women.

New research is showing that OA usually arises from being overweight and ignoring the need for exercise. Being 20 pounds or more overweight places a huge stress on cartilage in the knees, hips or spine. Over the years, failing to exercise weakens muscles that serve as shock absorbers around these joints, and poor nutrition also weakens bones and cartilage.

But the underlying cause of most OA is unresolved emotional stress. Instead of relieving stress with exercise, millions of Americans head for the refrigerator when they feel angry or frustrated, and they overeat snacks loaded with fat and sugar. For them, food has become a tranquilizer. And the standard American diet, equally high in fat and sugar, only piles on more pounds that will eventually degrade and destroy cartilage in the knees, hips and spine.

All in all, 37 million Americans—or one in every seven—currently has some form of rheumatic disease. Meanwhile, RA and OA cause more disability and financial loss than any other common ailments.

Do You Really Have Arthritis?

When Aunt Jane feels a twinge of pain in her neck, she may complain that her "arthritis" is acting up. Like most people with occasional joint pains, Aunt Jane has no idea whether her "arthritis" is actually RA or OA or whether it's even arthritis at all. Joint pain and stiffness are symptoms of several common diseases and infections that have nothing to do with arthritis.

The most common symptoms of arthritis are early morning stiffness, recurring tenderness or pain in any joint, swelling or obvious warmth and redness in one or more joints, and unexplained weight loss, weakness or fever combined with joint pain. If any of these symptoms persist for two weeks or longer, you may have some form of arthritis, and you should make an appointment to see your doctor for a diagnosis.

If you're really serious about overcoming arthritis, you *must* know exactly which type of arthritis you have. This means that your symptoms must be diagnosed by a physician. A medical diagnosis is essential to screen out several rare but dangerous forms of arthritis. Instead of arthritis, your doctor may find you have an infection, which can be easily cured with an antibiotic. Or she may find you have a severe case of RA, which requires immediate and aggressive treatment to prevent damage to cartilage and bone. Without knowing which type of arthritis you have, you could use an inappropriate Arthritis Fighter. For instance, an alternative therapy which may benefit RA could possibly worsen OA.

Virtually every rheumatologist (doctors who specialize in arthritis) agrees that mainstream medicine should be the first line of treatment for any type of arthritis. While drugs remain the core of medical treatment, most doctors also prescribe rest, exercise, heat and cold treatment and the use of splints to immobilize painful joints.

Generally, drugs for OA are milder and cause fewer problems. But drugs prescribed for RA and other autoimmune-induced arthritis can be highly toxic and cause serious side effects.

For autoimmune-induced arthritis, treatment begins with first-line drugs such as NSAIDs (Non-Steroid Anti-Inflammatory Drugs), which are analgesics like aspirin and ibuprofen. These drugs reduce both pain and inflammation. But, to be effective, as many as 16 aspirin tablets must be taken each day. Such large doses may lead to gastrointestinal bleeding and tinnitus, a ringing in the ears. Steroids, notorious for their side effects, are also occasionally prescribed as first-line drugs.

NSAIDs work by inhibiting prostaglandin production. But lack of prostaglandin may damage the lining of the stomach and intestines, allowing bleeding ulcers to form. Records show that one older person in four who takes daily doses of NSAIDs develops ulcers. Physicians frequently respond by prescribing a second drug to prevent ulcer formation. But these anti-ulcer drugs also have such side effects as abdominal pain and diarrhea.

The Grim Side Effects of Second-Line Arthritis Drugs

When NSAIDs lose their effectiveness, more powerful second-line drugs are prescribed. Classified as disease remittive drugs, these may include gold salts and antimalarial or immunosuppressive medications. Currently, for example, the most popular combination is a cocktail of methotrexate with antimalarial agents and cortisone.

Second-line drugs are prescribed primarily to modify severe RA and to increase the possibility of a remission. However, most are slow-acting, and it may take several months for benefits to appear.

Depending on the drug, between 15 and 30 percent of patients find side effects so intolerable that their doctor must switch them to another medication. Physicians often spend considerable time juggling with combinations of second-line drugs to find a tolerable balance between maximum benefits and minimum side effects.

Among side effects reported by users of second-line drugs are anemia, bone marrow suppression and nausea, borderline diabetes, headache, high cholesterol, hypertension, impaired immunity, kidney and liver overload or damage, loss of appetite, nutritional deficiencies, muscle weakness or skin rashes with itching. Any side effects must be carefully monitored by a physician throughout the time you are taking a drug. This could be years. All this can cost a hefty sum, especially if you're taking gold injections.

But whether you take aspirin or gold injections, drugs work only on a single biological pathway. They cannot restore strength to weakened muscles, increase the range of motion of a joint or transform depression and hopelessness into optimism and hope. All are essential before you can fully recover from arthritis.

Give Orthodox Medicine a Fair Shot First

Despite the drawbacks of drugs, I strongly urge you to consult a physician if you have arthritis symptoms and to follow any treatment your physician prescribes. For people who lack the motivation or commitment to adopt our Arthritis Fighters, medical treatment is the only option.

I do not endorse, recommend or encourage you to stop continuing your medical treatment without consulting your doctor first. This book is not intended to challenge medical treatment but to complement it. My intention is that the Arthritis Fighters are for use in conjunction with medical treatment and not as an alternative. This provides a true whole-person approach that will boost your chances of recovery.

All this implies, of course, that you should have your doctor's approval before you adopt and use any of the Arthritis Fighter techniques in this book. Your doctor's close cooperation is also necessary because, if drugs don't appear to help you while our Arthritis Fighters are obviously beneficial, you may not wish to continue taking the drugs.

We're talking about a gray area here because if you are using both drugs and Arthritis Fighter techniques and your arthritis improves, your doctor is almost sure to claim that the drugs are responsible.

If there's any doubt, stop using the Arthritis Fighters for a while. Should the arthritis symptoms worsen, this strongly suggests that the Arthritis Fighters were providing the benefit. Test results may occasionally be fogged by periodic flare-ups or remissions. But if several tests clearly show that your medication isn't helping, you could ask your doctor to change or reduce the dosage or eliminate it altogether.

Don't Let Drugs Become a Medical Dead End

In severe cases of immune-induced arthritis, you may have to keep on taking a maintenance drug. But in most milder cases or in OA or possibly gout, the Arthritis Fighter techniques may make it unnecessary to continue taking drugs. It's well to remember that a drug can only do what a healthy body-mind can do for itself. Once your level of wellness improves, drug treatment may no longer be required.

That is something only your doctor can decide. If your doctor believes in medicalizing everything and solving every problem with drugs, she may automatically veto any alternative therapy you wish to try. Some doctors still admit only grudgingly that exercise or heat and cold therapy can be helpful, despite both being endorsed by the Arthritis Foundation. Such an attitude strongly discourages you from exploring any option outside drug therapy.

In such case, your doctor could be doing you a real disservice. One solution is to change to another doctor who realizes that drugs and surgery are not the only ways to get well. I suggest choosing a doctor who is familiar with other branches of medicine such as behavioral and preventive medicine and psychoneuroimmunology. Though these may sound unfamiliar, they are recognized branches of medicine staffed by highly trained M.D.s, psychiatrists, physiatrists, neurologists and nutritionists with top credentials from leading medical schools.

While they may prescribe drugs or surgery if really essential, these doctors prefer to rely on nondrug therapies similar to those of our Arthritis Fighters. Hundreds of doctors have transferred to these fields after becoming disenchanted with the disappointing results and overuse of many drug and surgical procedures.

In fact, most of the Arthritis Fighter techniques in this book were developed by researchers working in behavioral or preventive medicine or in the science of psychoneuroimmunology. Some of their discoveries are causing mainstream medical researchers to completely rethink their approach to arthritis.

Is Science Looking Down the Wrong End of the Microscope?

Virtually all the research efforts of mainstream medicine seem targeted towards explaining arthritis in terms of molecular biology. This implies that arthritis must have a physical or a mechanical cause such as a toxin, virus, bacteria, injury, a joint misalignment or a dysfunctional gene. This is because in our materialistic, profit-driven society, researchers are locked into seeking a cure for arthritis in the form of a chemical agent. Once found, this chemical can then be mass-produced and sold at a huge profit by the pharmaceutical industry. Thus far, no real cure for arthritis has ever been discovered. And considering the complexity of each type of arthritis, it is highly unlikely that one ever will.

The problem with this approach is that it totally ignores the role of any psychological or emotional component in the arthritis process. That's because the drug industry cannot make a pill that will change the beliefs and thoughts in our minds. And it is largely the way we think that is responsible for the stress that sets off arthritis.

Arthritis: A Physical Disease That Begins in the Mind

Medical science claims that the cause of arthritis is unknown. But many indications clearly point to stress as the underlying cause. Consider, for example, these facts recently reported in medical studies and journals.

"Fibrositis appears to be caused by tension, anxiety, hostility and frustration. . . . Lupus and RA flare-ups are frequently triggered by emotional upsets. . . . When emotional and physical stresses are relieved, many people notice that their RA improves. . . . Stress aggravates arthritis pain, especially in people with RA. . . . Stress often triggers a gout attack."

"RA pain increases in direct proportion to the stress in a person's life. The pain then causes more stress, ad infinitum."

"Lower back pain is frequently triggered by stress which causes muscles in the back to go into spasm. The slightest strain, such as raising a window, can then cause a microscopic muscle tear, setting off an excruciating pain in the back."

"Norman Cousins recovered from ankylosing spondylitis, a life-threatening collagen disease, by spending several hours each day laughing at comedy films. Since then, others have used the same method to laugh away RA and other forms of autoimmune arthritis."

These reports show that our mood is intimately linked to our immune system and to our inner healing powers, and that if a cure for arthritis exists, it is more likely to be found between our ears than in our joints.

Meanwhile, a plethora of new findings from the rapidly

growing science of psychoneuroimmunology is providing intriguing proof of the body's inner healing powers to relieve the pain and symptoms of arthritic disease.

What Exactly Are Behavioral and Preventive Medicine and Psychoneuroimmunology?

- *Behavioral medicine* is a branch of medical science based on the idea that we can change the way we feel by changing the way we act (or behave). By breathing deeply and slowly, for example, while we focus the mind on a single thought, we can quickly become so relaxed that our sensitivity to pain is significantly diminished.
- *Preventive medicine* is a branch of medical science designed to prevent infectious and chronic disease. By replacing meat with fish, eating lots of fruits and vegetables, exercising regularly and not smoking, we can cut the risk of ever getting heart disease, stroke, cancer, hypertension, diabetes and even arthritis by up to 90 percent.
- *Psychoneuroimmunology* is the study of the mind's link to the body's immune system and healing mechanisms. Our nervous and endocrine systems are constantly communicating our moods and feelings to our immune system. For example, laughter and a positive attitude enhance immunity and boost our inner healing powers while grief, loss or depression weaken both our immune system and our body's healing mechanisms.

The Best Nondrug Way to Recover from Arthritis

Recent research in each of these fields has identified what we shall henceforth call the body's healing-regeneration system. No one claims it will restore damaged cartilage, but

13

our healing-regeneration system may well offer the best non-drug way to recover from any form of arthritis. Most Arthritis Fighters in this book are self-help strategies through which we can also access our own innate power to create and restore health and well-being.

Self-healing is based on the concept that, with the exception of a few virulent diseases such as AIDS, rabies or cancer, when the cause of disease is removed, the body becomes a self-healing entity. For example, when a coronary artery is partially blocked with fatty plaque, it is not necessarily blocked for good. Extensive research by Dean Ornish, M.D. and others has demonstrated that when we remove the fat and cholesterol from our diet, which is the cause of the disease, and when we begin to exercise and get the stress out of our life, the artery may begin to clear itself.

The body is not a machine made of metal and plastic. Every part of it consists of living cells. In many cases, our cells will regenerate to heal and restore a damaged body part. Dental cavities won't regenerate, but broken bones will. Cartilage damaged by arthritis is difficult to restore, but the muscles that cushion that cartilage can be restored, as can much of the joint's original range of motion.

The Arthritis Fighters in this book place powerful healing tools in your hands through which you can access many of the body's self-healing powers. No proof exists, but strong indications point to our healing-regeneration system as the real source of any long-term remission from autoimmune arthritis.

This isn't to say that Arthritis Fighters will cure arthritis or totally relieve every last vestige of stiffness or pain. But if you're really sincere about beating arthritis without the side effects of drugs, there's an excellent chance you *can* decrease the frequency and intensity of arthritis pain and symptoms.

And you *can* reduce them to levels that can easily be tolerated.

Every one of us has the ability to tap into our inner healing powers. Before you can access them, however, you must first learn to communicate with your body through the Eight Vital Ways to Activate Your Body's Inner Healing Powers in Chapter 2.

CHAPTER TWO

Arthritis Relief from Within: Eight Vital Ways to Activate Your Body's Inner Healing Powers

Our healing-regeneration system is a powerful psychobiological mechanism through which a positive belief or emotion can be translated into physical healing. It begins with the beliefs that we hold in our minds, and it includes the nervous and endocrine systems and our immune system. All its mechanisms function on a very subtle level.

Our healing-regeneration system is key to beating arthritis.

But the body's recuperative system cannot be accessed directly. Instead, we must use an indirect approach.

Let me explain. Whether it functions on the physical, psychological or nutritional level, each Arthritis Fighter has an emotional component through which we can tap into our inner healing system. For instance, the benefits of exercise are due as much to the emotional component of exercise as to the actual exercise itself. Whenever we use any Arthritis Fighter technique, we create an emotional byproduct that indirectly turns on all or part of our inner healing powers.

The eight steps below describe how we can use new knowledge, attitudes, perception and strategies to tap into our inner healing powers whenever we use the Arthritis Fighters in this book.

ARTHRITIS FIGHTER #1: The Eight Vital Recovery Steps That Unlock Your Inner Healing Powers

---

STEP 1: ACTIVATE YOUR PLACEBO EFFECT

Whenever a doctor gives a sugar pill to any group of people with RA and tells them it is a "medically proven joint pain reducing agent," at least 30 percent of the group will begin to feel better in just a short time. Their improvement springs from a mechanism in the mind called the "placebo effect." The placebo effect arises from a person's faith, belief and expectation in the healing power of a therapy rather than from the therapy itself.

The power of suggestion has a tremendous effect on anyone with arthritis. In fact, RA has the highest placebo remission rate of any medical condition.

In almost every person with arthritis, having something to believe in is all they need to unlock their intrinsic healing power. Researchers have discovered that a strong belief is often a more powerful healer than many drugs. Almost 50 percent of people who believe they will recover from arthritis do get better, even if the improvement is only temporary.

Careful studies show that the placebo effect improves a person's chance of recovery from almost any nonfatal disease or injury—and also from surgery—by an average of 33 percent. But the improvement rate jumps to 40 to 60 percent or more when patients are given a detailed explanation of their disease and told how their therapy intervenes in the disease process. Knowing exactly how everything works makes it much easier to believe in.

For example, to prepare a group of patients for bypass surgery, doctors in one large hospital carefully explained the function of the cardiovascular system and how the operation would restore blood supply to the heart. Before the operation, each patient had a thorough understanding of the modus operandi of both the disease and the operation.

But when the group was given heart function tests following the operation, results revealed that only 20 percent of patients showed any physical improvement. Yet 75 percent of the patients reported feeling greatly improved, and many showed significant improvement in exercise stress tests.

Obviously, 55 percent of the group's reported improvement was due directly to the placebo effect. This was much higher than the 33 percent rate expected. This led doctors to conclude that the more a person knows and understands about the way her disease and treatment functions, the more likely she is to believe it will work.

Mind as Medicine

To turn on your own placebo effect at maximum power, you need only read and absorb the facts in this book. Once you understand the arthritis process and how each Arthritis Fighter functions, you will find it much easier to believe in your therapy and to build a strong expectation in its ability to succeed.

So great is the power of the placebo effect that many therapies work that shouldn't. For example, a strong belief in a worthless therapy may result in a 33 percent improvement. For generations, hucksters have peddled worthless nostrums and unproven remedies that they claimed would cure arthritis. That some actually worked is entirely due to the placebo effect.

Believe in the ability of anything to heal arthritis—be it snake or bee venom, injections of fetal lamb cells, magnets, vibrators, gin-soaked raisins or pulverized fish cartilage—and your arthritis is likely to improve. The extent of your improvement will be approximately equal to the benefit that you expect to receive.

It may be appropriate here to caution you to guard your wallet. Since no proven cure exists at this time, arthritis is a fertile field for quack remedies and hucksters. Currently, the National Institutes of Health Office of Alternative Medicine is investigating a variety of unproven remedies for arthritis. But their tests are hampered by the placebo effect.

The pain and discomfort of arthritis lead at least one American in three to try an unproven arthritis remedy each year. Many cures are reported, arising not only from the placebo effect but from two other reasons. First, because no medical diagnosis was ever made and the person did not have genuine arthritis in the first place. And second, because the person took medical treatment before trying the unproven remedy. Eventually, the medical treatment kicked in and worked.

While it's true that absolute proof of the efficacy of some of our Arthritis Fighters has never been demonstrated by clinical trials, many have been documented in professional journals, while others have shown promise in smaller studies.

A good way to size up the probable worth of any arthritis treatment is to ask whether it is active or passive. Active therapies like exercise, visualization or stress management techniques all require you to take an active role in your own recovery by making use of your muscles or mind. Frequently, active therapies are much more successful than passive therapies in which you swallow a pill or have something done to you by someone else while you do nothing. In any case, be especially careful about handing over money for arthritis treatment in Mexico. And be aware that dubious treatments are sometimes promoted by medical doctors in the United States as well.

The Tremendous Healing Power of Suggestion

Millennia ago, witch doctors and shamans discovered that the remedy they used was less important than the attitude they could arouse in their patients. Through much of human history, professional healers have used rituals and symbols like wooden masks, rattles and animal sacrifices to promote the placebo effect in people who were sick.

Though doctors try to disparage the placebo effect, for millions of Americans the hospital is now the temple of healing, the doctor in the white coat is the high priest, and the bottle of pills is the modern-day symbol of healing. Recent research suggests that a large proportion of the benefit from any drug or surgical treatment may actually be derived from the placebo effect.

Doctors often consider the placebo effect a nuisance when testing drugs. In every clinical trial, the action of the placebo effect must be added to the action of the drug when measuring results. In many trials, especially on patients with RA, tests show that the placebo effect provides greater benefit than the drug's pharmaceutical action.

As a result, many doctors consider that the placebo effect contaminates the pharmaceutical benefit of their drugs. They are apt to be embarrassed when a patient's belief in an unproven therapy leads to improvement. Somehow, because the placebo effect can't be turned on by a marketable drug, it isn't good medicine. Doctors also point out that the healing power of the placebo effect is often temporary.

Exorcise Your Arthritis with the Placebo Effect

That may be your doctor's view. But as far as you're concerned, whether your arthritis is improved by a drug or by the placebo effect, what difference does it make? Whatever causes your arthritis to improve is good medicine. If the placebo effect can relieve your arthritis pain and symptoms, isn't that better than taking some toxic drug with adverse side effects?

Undoubtedly, the placebo effect is your body-mind's most powerful tool for healing arthritis. To help activate it, I recommend, first, that you base your recovery program on the Arthritis Fighters in this book and that you avoid the more outlandish and unproven fringe remedies. It makes more sense to generate your placebo effect by believing in a therapy that works rather than believing in something as dubious as carrying radioactive rocks in your pocket.

Second, you can keep your placebo effect permanently alive by continuing to use the therapies you believe in. Once their arthritis symptoms disappear, all too many people stop

21

exercising, visualizing or practicing whatever Arthritis Fighters they may have been using. Since your placebo effect depends on having a therapy to believe in, it can continue to flourish only for as long as you keep practicing that therapy. Once you stop using a therapy you believe in, your placebo effect evaporates and back comes your arthritis.

Third, be sure to boost your placebo effect by learning and understanding everything you can about the arthritis process and about the therapies you are using. If you forget the rationale behind your therapies, refresh your knowledge and keep it alive.

Fourth, the placebo effect works synergistically with all the other steps that open our inner healing powers. Each of our steps reinforces the others. By continuing to use the other steps, your placebo effect will remain permanently strong and powerful and will not fade with the passage of time.

STEP 2: BECOME A MEDICALLY INFORMED LAYPERSON

The literature is filled with case histories of people who achieved a significant level of control over arthritis pain by learning all there is to know about it. At least one series of documented studies confirms that you can help conquer arthritis pain by simply understanding more about the disease.

When Dr. Kate Lorig of Stanford University studied a group of 224 arthritis patients, she found that educating them about their disorder was as effective in reducing pain as any of the most popular arthritis medications. During the 4-year study, members of the test group who received the instruction made 43 percent fewer visits to a doctor than did members of the control group who received no arthritis education.

A basic principle of all self-healing is to learn as much as possible about your disorder. Without this know-how you might apply heat to a joint when you should be applying cold, or you might exercise when you should be resting. Being well informed about arthritis also helps you work as a partner with your doctor, and it helps you to make intelligent choices and decisions about medical treatment.

Chapter 3 supplies a clear, scientifically based explanation of the arthritis process, while the description of each Arthritis Fighter expands your knowledge. This information gives you a new understanding of the arthritis process and how you can intervene in it yourself to a greater extent than your doctor can. You'll discover, for example, that each of us has a greater arsenal of arthritis fighting action-steps at our disposal than any physician.

A compelling reason to understand the arthritis process is that some of our Arthritis Fighters use techniques so new and innovative that many people, including physicians, may regard them with skepticism and disbelief. But by empowering yourself with know-how, you will swiftly see how these seemingly radical action-steps work to diminish pain and arthritis symptoms. Seeing is believing. And belief is all you need to turn on your placebo effect.

STEP 3: UNLEASH THE POWER OF YOUR ENABLING EFFECT

Two weeks after Betty began a series of daily exercises to improve the range of motion of her joints, her arthritis pain began to diminish. This improvement inspired Betty to add more exercises to her daily routine. It took only two additional weeks to restore almost normal flexibility to her hips, knees and elbows. By now, Betty felt so upbeat, she could hardly wait to begin using biofeedback, the next step in her personal program for beating arthritis.

Betty didn't know it, but as she attributed each success to her own efforts, she was empowering herself with formidable amounts of enabling effect. The "enabling effect" is the psychologists' term for the empowerment we experience whenever we attribute an improvement in our health to our own efforts rather than to a passive therapy, such as a drug or medical treatment, worked on us by someone else.

Studies show that the enabling effect is a powerful booster of the placebo effect. Take therapeutic imagery for arthritis as an example (AF#17).

1. When a person has full faith and belief in the healing power of therapeutic imagery, the placebo effect increases the effectiveness of that therapy by 33 percent.

2. When the person also has a complete understanding of the arthritis process and how imagery intervenes, its effectiveness is increased by approximately 50 percent.

3. But when the person begins to experience actual improvement from the imagery, the enabling effect kicks in and its total effectiveness soars by roughly 70 percent.

In other words, someone who has become a medically educated layperson, and who experiences both the placebo and enabling effects, receives 70 percent greater benefit from therapeutic imagery than a person who has done none of these things. The same thing is true whenever you use your mind or muscles to perform *any* active therapy that works.

Lick Arthritis with Constant Feedback

The secret to releasing this inner healing power is to provide yourself with constant feedback. For example, if we're using one or more of the Arthritis Fighters, and the pain level of our arthritis is steadily dropping week by week, that is all the feedback most of us need to keep our enabling effect turned on at maximum strength.

To harness the power of your enabling effect, whenever you adopt any Arthritis Fighter technique in this book:

1. Write down your arthritis-relief goal. That might be total relief from pain and stiffness.

2. Divide that goal into a series of small, easy-to-attain mini-goals.

3. Know that the success of achieving the first mini-goal empowers you to achieve the second mini-goal. As success breeds success, your enabling effect will propel you on to reach your third mini-goal, then your fourth, fifth and so on.

4. Make mini-goals that are relatively easy to reach. Suppose that on a scale from 1 to 10, you rate your level of arthritis pain and stiffness as 10. Instead of aiming for a target of 0 (complete remission), set a target of 9 as your first mini-goal. To reach this, you need to reduce your arthritis discomfort by only 10 percent. Such Arthritis Fighters as Heat and Cold Therapy (AF#2) or Exercise (AF#3) should achieve this mini-goal quite quickly. As you achieve this small step, the feedback you experience propels you on toward your next mini-goal, a pain level of 8.

By attributing success to your own efforts, your enabling effect spurs you on to reach ever-lower levels of stiffness and pain.

Each time you detect a noticeable improvement, it provides powerful confirmation that you have a great deal of control over your arthritis and that you yourself can often do as much or more to beat the disease than any drug or treatment given you by someone else.

To maintain positive feedback, I recommend keeping a diary. Only by keeping a daily record can you detect an often slow but gradual increase in your levels of comfort, ease and freedom of movement. Note the date and time of each event that seems related to your arthritis and use a scale from 1 to 10 to record the intensity of pain, stiffness, inflammation and so on. Note any circumstances or events that seem to precede flare-ups; the levels of stress you experience at home and at work; what you ate or drank prior to flare-ups; the side effects of any medications; and if you're female, any association with oral contraceptives or menstrual periods.

A well-kept diary like this is also an excellent diagnostic tool for your doctor.

STEP 4: UNLOCK YOUR BODY'S HEALING POWERS BY DOING SOMETHING ACTIVE

Therapies for arthritis are either active or passive. Passive therapies involve swallowing a drug or herb, receiving an injection or having something done to you by someone else while you do nothing. Passive therapies include taking medications, undergoing surgery or traction, taking ultrasound or acupuncture treatment or a musculoskeletal adjustment or massage and undergoing psychological analysis or counseling. Many passive therapies, including medical treatment such as knee arthroscopy, can be extremely beneficial. But others, especially drugs, are frequently ineffective for long-term relief of arthritis pain or symptoms. One reason is that by delegating responsibility for your arthritis pain to another person, or to a drug or other passive treatment, you create a dependency that may sabotage your body's own inner-healing mechanisms.

Active therapies, by contrast, force you to take a role in your own recovery and to look to yourself for relief from arthritis. Ranging from exercise to breathing techniques, relaxation training, biofeedback, heat and cold treatment, yoga and stretching, upgrading your diet, using therapeutic imagery or cutting out smoking, action therapies all force you to become actively involved in beating your arthritis.

Each of the Arthritis Fighters in this book is an active therapy that has been demonstrated to provide real physical or mental benefit. Whenever you use an Arthritis Fighter action-step, you express a powerful belief in your ability to recover from arthritis. This belief automatically accesses your body's inner healing powers each time you use an Arthritis Fighter action-step. These other mind-body effects may double, triple or even quadruple the benefit of the Arthritis Fighter action-step itself.

With the exception of the placebo effect, our other healing-regeneration powers are difficult to access through passive therapies. Only by acting to help ourselves can we unlock the awesome power of our enabling and endorphin effects and the body's other healing-regeneration mechanisms.

To activate these powerful built-in healing powers, we have to act. To get results we have to use our mind and muscles to do what it takes to succeed in overcoming arthritis. This book can't stretch or exercise or visualize for you. It puts you in the driver's seat and it's up to you to act.

So if your physician or other health professional isn't able to help, your willingness to act and help yourself may often do more to relieve your arthritis than any drug or doctor can.

STEP 5: DON'T LET COMPLACENCY SABOTAGE YOUR INNER HEALING POWERS

Mary was 60 pounds overweight and suffered from OA in the knees, hips and spine. She was also plagued by chronic indigestion and constipation. Since she lived close by, I let her read an early draft of this book.

She returned it a week later and said proudly, "You'll be glad to know I've switched over to low-fat cookies and I'm adding bran to my diet."

That was it. Nothing about eating more fruits and vegetables, losing weight or beginning to exercise. As I finished this book three months later, Mary's constipation had improved. But she was still seriously overweight and her OA and chronic indigestion had actually worsened.

Token cooperation with our Arthritis Fighters isn't enough to beat arthritis. I've had people read this book and say, "That's all very nice and I'm sure it's true, but it wouldn't work for me. I prefer to go on living the way I am."

Most of our Arthritis Fighters do call for a change in attitude, diet and lifestyle. And most people who have arthritis have been living and eating unwisely for so many years that they are resistant and reluctant to change. So they continue to rely on drugs to relieve their arthritis pain and symptoms. This allows them to continue with the same counterproductive habits that caused their arthritis in the first place.

If you're really sincere about liberating yourself from arthritis, you cannot afford to be locked into this vicious circle of complacency. *It can totally block and immobilize your body's inner-healing system.* Fortunately, there *is* something you can do about it. The core principle of behavorial medicine tells us that we can change the way we feel by changing the way we act.

If you lack the motivation to act, you can boost your motivation by acting first. Where motivation is concerned, the mind is like an old-fashioned water pump. Before it will pump water, you have to prime it with water first. The mind works the same way. To mobilize the motivation to act, you have to act first. Then the motivation will come.

How to Handle Lack of Motivation

If you lack motivation to walk around the block, just forget about motivation and walk around the block. Just doing it will boost your self-esteem, and you'll feel so good that you'll be motivated to do it again.

We feel good because we've broken the vicious circle of complacency that has frozen our body's built-in pain-relief and healing mechanisms. For many of us, complacency may be all that is stopping us from recovering from arthritis.

Liberate Yourself from This Insidious Arthritis Trap

Psychologists have discovered that the only thing that keeps us complacent is the desire to remain in our "comfort zone." To offset the stress of growing up, most of us create a lifestyle built around watching TV, eating sweet and fatty foods and avoiding most forms of physical exertion. Together, these indulgences comprise our "comfort zone."

29

Eating, for example, is such a nurturing and comforting social experience that we continue to eat the same foods that we grew up with. This learned behavior becomes a deeply engrained part of our lives. As we reach adulthood, eating foods high in sugar, fat and animal protein continues to be comforting because it reinforces memories of when we were fed these same comfort foods as youngsters. So we call it "the good life." But our "good life" is often the direct cause of OA and gout, and it can also worsen RA.

As we grow older, we continue to rely on these same rich foods to tranquilize us against the stresses of modern life. By our mid-20s, we so crave being in the "comfort zone" that most of us assume we are locked into these habits for life.

Millions of us probably have some idea of how to eat and exercise to improve arthritis. But we still don't do it. The result is that most physicians accept the stereotyped assumption that Americans are weak-willed, self-indulgent people who waver easily, yield to every temptation and would rather watch TV than do gentle exercises that could relieve their arthritis. So doctors continue to prescribe drugs instead of natural therapies.

There's certainly some truth to that. But, frankly, I don't buy into that popular image. In recent years, over 30 million Americans have quit smoking cigarettes, an accomplishment more difficult than adopting all the Arthritis Fighters in this book at once.

Behavorial psychologists soon learned why people succeed at quitting smoking. It's because those who give up smoking see a tremendous improvement in their health and well-being in just a few days.

To boost our motivation, we need almost immediate feedback. Numerous studies have shown that people with arthritis *are* willing to change their diet and lifestyle, provided they see an improvement in their arthritis in a matter of days.

Positive feedback in the form of a decrease in arthritis pain and symptoms is almost certain when you adopt and use the Arthritis Fighters in this book. Granted, some produce results faster than others. But observations show that almost everyone who begins to use these natural techniques soon begins to feel tremendously better.

When this happens, your enabling effect kicks in and the healing process is almost identical to that described in Step 3, "Lick Arthritis with Constant Feedback." So turn back to Step 3 and learn how diary keeping and mini-goals can provide you with almost constant positive feedback. For most of us, success is all the motivation we need to step out of our comfort zone and conquer our complacency.

STEP 6: TURN ON YOUR BRAIN'S FEEL-GOOD MECHANISM

Marjorie had been a jogger for years. Then she tore the cartilage in her knee and had to stop. Almost immediately, Marjorie began to feel depressed. Her doctor prescribed an antidepressant drug. But the drug produced such uncomfortable side effects that Marjorie stopped taking it.

Looking back, Marjorie realized why the depression had hit. It was because she had stopped running. After an arthroscopy operation on her knee, Marjorie was able to begin a program of brisk daily walking and her depression vanished. Once she had jogged to stay fit and slim, but now Marjorie is walking so that she can feel good once again.

"Runner's high" is the popular name for the feel-good mechanism that lifted Marjorie's spirits. It's an incredible feeling of well-being that suppresses the experience of pain and stabilizes the emotions for the rest of the day. Exercise physiologists know that runner's high is due to the release of endorphins in the brain.

After 35 minutes or so of brisk rhythmic exercise, the brain releases clouds of tiny peptide molecules called "endorphins." These are natural morphine-like opiates that switch off pain by binding on to pain receptors in the brain. In the process, they wipe out depression and anxiety, and they boost self-esteem and build a strong self-image that lasts until bedtime.

Like Marjorie, tens of thousands of Americans with arthritis know better than to sit on the couch watching television. Instead, they lace on their walking shoes and step out briskly for 35 minutes or more. Those who can't walk pedal a stationary bicycle, while others swim or exercise in water.

The Body's Natural Narcotics Deaden Pain

Almost any type of rhythmic exercise can elevate mood. You don't have to run or jog. Begin with a low-intensity exercise like walking 3 to 4 times a week for up to 30 minutes, if you can. Then as your fitness improves, gradually work up to where you can walk (or swim or bicycle) for 35 minutes at a brisk pace. That means a pace sufficiently fast to speed up your breathing and heart rate and, swimming excepted, to cause mild perspiration to appear on your brow in warm weather.

Proof of endorphins' ability to reduce arthritis pain was confirmed in a study by Martha Storandt, Ph.D. (reported in the *Journal of Gerontology*, 1995). After examining 87 healthy people aged 60 to 73 who participated in a year-long program of rhythmic and flexibility exercise training, Dr. Storandt found that not only does exercise release endorphins, but it boosts our sense of well-being, self-esteem, self-confidence and morale, while also slowing or reversing physical and psychological decline due to such degenerative diseases as arthritis.

Meanwhile, no improvement was observed in a control group of 34 people who did not exercise. These results led Dr. Storandt to suggest that exercise for older people should be as routine as brushing their teeth.

We can also turn on our feel-good mechanism without exercising. Several double blind studies have found that endorphins are responsible for pain relief due to the placebo effect. When study participants were given placebos and told they were powerful pain-killers, approximately 33 percent experienced a significant reduction in pain. Study authors concluded that analgesia due to the placebo effect is entirely due to production of endorphins in the brain.

Researchers also discovered that the average amount of pain relief due to placebo endorphin release is equivalent to receiving 8 mgs of real morphine. Undoubtedly, exercise provides pain relief equivalent to still greater amounts of real morphine.

But placebo studies have clearly demonstrated that endorphins *can* also be released by such mild activities as practicing yoga (AF#4) or using relaxation training (AF#16). So if you're unable to do any kind of rhythmic exercise at all, stretching or relaxation may be other ways to access the giant pain-killer that lurks in your mind.

Yet rhythmic exercise is still the surest way to tap into the pain-relieving power of your brain. And whether you exercise in water or pedal a stationary bicycle in the living room, most people with arthritis *are* able to exercise.

So try it for yourself—with your doctor's permission, of course. Then compare the powerful feeling of accomplishment that you experience with the feeling of helplessness and passivity that frequently accompanies dependence on drug medication.

STEP 7. HOPE IS GOOD MEDICINE FOR ARTHRITIS

When Melanie told a friend she had arthritis, the friend advised that there was nothing Melanie could do. She'd just have to learn to live with it.

Such advice causes people with arthritis to give up hope and resign themselves to the belief that nothing can be done. Believing this, Melanie put off seeing a doctor for months. The delay merely aggravated the cartilage damage in her right knee. When Melanie finally did see a doctor, he told her it was just in time. Any further delay could have led to permanent crippling.

Suggestion plays a tremendous role in arthritis recovery. A negative suggestion that you must learn to live with arthritis and take drugs for life can be far more crippling than the disease itself. Studies show that people who have strong hope and strongly positive attitudes, and who firmly believe they will get well, recover 25 to 50 percent faster from almost any type of nonfatal disease than someone with a passive, helpless attitude.

In a study at the University of Alabama on 65 patients with OA of the hip and knee, researchers subjected each participant to a battery of psychological tests and then analyzed every factor in their lifestyles. They then X-rayed each patient for joint damage and related these factors to the extent of pain experienced by each person.

When the results were pooled, it was found that the extent of pain and disability experienced by each participant was far more closely related to their outlook and attitude than to any physical damage or discomfort caused by the arthritis. Those patients who felt the highest levels of hopelessness and helplessness experienced the highest levels of pain and disability. Researchers concluded that a cheerful outlook and high hopes for recovery could work wonders in reducing arthritis pain and disability.

These findings were confirmed in the 1980s when Albert Bandura, Ph.D. of Stanford University discovered that arthritis pain was aggravated by feelings of hopelessness and helplessness. When Bandura taught a group of arthritis patients to ease their symptoms with exercise and other natural techniques, almost all experienced less pain and increased mobility. But it wasn't merely the exercise and other therapies that led to pain relief. Researchers found that most of the benefit was due to a change in the patients' attitude. Instead of feeling hopeless and depressed, they now felt in control of their life and health.

Then Bandura designed a similar but larger study. Results showed that 35 percent of participants reported a decrease in pain, 20 percent had improvement in joint mobility and 18 percent experienced a decrease in depression. Bandura called this "self-efficacy."

The Therapeutic Power of Hope

Mobilizing self-efficacy is largely a matter of mobilizing hope. Accept that you have arthritis. Then accept that, with very few exceptions, no disease is totally incurable. There's no such thing as false hope.

But hope must be realistic. I don't pin any real hopes on

35

copper bracelets, bee venom or other unproved nostrums. The Arthritis Foundation warns that false hopes raised by quack cures can lead to depression when the cure fails. (While this may be true, it overlooks the fact that medical treatment may also fail.)

The principal benefit of our Arthritis Fighters is to instill hope. Without hope, self-efficacy cannot be mobilized. You may not recover completely, but you should be able to manage your arthritis to the point where most pain and symptoms fade away.

Hope is good medicine for arthritis sufferers. Hope enables us to see arthritis as a challenge to be overcome rather than as a hopeless dysfunction we must learn to live with for the rest of our lives.

Herbert Benson, M.D. of Harvard Medical School puts it another way. He recommends becoming an "exceptional patient." For instance, if the statistical odds of recovery from RA are only 1 in 10 each year, using our Arthritis Fighters may well help you to become that exceptional one person who makes a spontaneous and complete recovery.

STEP 8: TREAT THE WHOLE PERSON INSTEAD OF JUST THE PART THAT HURTS

Gout can be helped by diet. But it takes exercise, weight loss and a change in attitude to effectively overcome it for good.

As with all forms of arthritis, results are best when we put the combined powers of body, mind and nutrition to work to access our healing-regeneration system on three different levels.

This threefold approach to healing is also known as "holistic or whole-person healing." When we use one or more Arthritis Fighters that work on the physical level, one or more that work on the psychological level, and one or more that work on the nutritional level, we are using a holistic approach to overcoming arthritis. This multilevel approach lets us communicate with our healing system in a language it can understand.

Arthritis is a whole-person dysfunction, so it takes a whole-person approach to overcome it.

For example, any type of exercise, from working out with weights to rhythmic exercises like walking or swimming, to yoga stretching and deep breathing, not only benefits us physically, but it boosts our self-esteem. In turn, our heightened self-esteem enhances every aspect of our healing-regeneration system.

Walking briskly for 35 minutes, or swimming or bicycling, releases endorphins in the brain that reduce the intensity of arthritis pain and lift our spirits for the rest of the day. Every physical Arthritis Fighter has an emotional component that helps restore balance to the entire body-mind.

Likewise, every mental action has a profound effect on the physical body. Arthritis Fighters that function on the psychological level—such as laughter, biofeedback, belief restructuring and therapeutic imagery—induce a variety of physical effects ranging from muscle relaxation to relief of tension and strengthening of the immune system.

We can also access our natural healing powers by using relaxation techniques to calm and restore balance to the entire body-mind. Nutritional Arthritis Fighters also help activate our healing-regeneration system. As we lose weight and feel better, we become more cheerful and optimistic. And researchers in the field of psychoneuroimmunology discovered long ago that positive thoughts and feelings boost our inner-healing powers, while negative thoughts and feelings suppress them.

Maximize Your Body's Recuperative Powers with a Holistic Approach

To use holistic healing, simply select one or more Arthritis Fighters from each of the following levels and combine them in an overall program to beat arthritis.

Physical Action-Steps: AF#2, 3, 4, 5, 6 and 7
Nutritional Action-Steps: AF#8, 9, 10, 11, 12, 13 and 14
Psychological Action-Steps: AF#15, 16, 17 and 18

For example, a combination of exercise, laughter, plant-based diet, relaxation training and therapeutic imagery works on your fears, beliefs and emotions as much as your joints. When used in a bold combination like this, each Arthritis Fighter works synergistically to reinforce the others. This makes the total benefit far greater than the sum of the benefits of each individual Arthritis Fighter alone.

By empowering our healing-regeneration system on every level, these recovery steps demonstrate the need to broaden our view of arthritis beyond mere physical factors. They also provide tangible evidence that we do have control over our body and mind and that we are no longer helpless victims of arthritis.

CHAPTER THREE

Understanding Arthritis Is Key to Relief

One of the best ways to reduce the pain and symptoms of arthritis is to learn more about this disorder. For proof, we have only to look at a study made at Stanford University in 1986. In the study, 129 people aged 23 to 94—all with OA or RA—attended educational sessions about arthritis during a four-month period. The courses explained the disease process, and participants were taught to use natural therapies such as exercise and relaxation training to relieve pain.

Meanwhile, a control group of 61 participants was told to do the same exercise and relaxation therapies but without instruction about the arthritis process. After four months, the test group reported a decrease in pain more than double that of the control group. This study so clearly demonstrated the power of knowledge in reducing arthritis pain and symptoms that the Arthritis Foundation subsequently sponsored a nationwide arthritis education program.

This chapter presents a similar education program, complete with all the latest insights into the arthritis process. For example, the more you know about arthritis, the less frightening and mysterious it becomes. Understanding how arthritis functions helps you maintain your placebo effect at full strength. And it allows you to intervene successfully in the arthritis process.

I warn you, though. This chapter may sound like pure science fiction. As it unfolds, you will learn how RA arises out of the incessant cell wars that rage constantly within your body as legions of defenders fight on invisible battlegrounds to protect you against cancer and infectious diseases. Yet, it's all absolutely factual. And while you don't need to remember every last detail, you should at least have a basic understanding of the mechanisms in your body that lead up to arthritis.

UNDERSTANDING THE GENESIS OF ARTHRITIS

Let's begin by taking a look at the joints in our bodies. A joint is any place where two bones meet and our joint mechanisms allow us to turn, twist, bend and move. Spinal vertebrae are a series of strong joints that permit relatively little movement. Hips and shoulders have ball and socket joints that permit them to rotate. Knee and wrist joints are more flexible but more easily damaged.

Each joint consists of connective tissue and includes tendons, ligaments and cartilage that support the bones and keep them aligned. Tendons are tough, ropelike tissues that attach muscles to bones. Ligaments are other strong, cordlike tissues that wrap around joints and connect bones to each other. Bursa are fluid-filled sacs that cushion bones, tendons and ligaments and prevent them from having contact with each other.

Cartilage is a smooth, tough, resilient, elastic layer of shock-absorbing tissue that covers the end of every bone in every joint. Cartilage is so incredibly smooth that it glides without friction against any other piece of cartilage. Without protective pads of cartilage, bone would grind against bone in our joints.

All these components—the entire joint in fact—are enclosed inside a thin capsule called the "synovium" (also known as the "synovial membrane" or "inner lining.") The synovium exists to hold in the synovial fluid, a joint lubricant that is secreted into the joint whenever joint movement begins.

Additionally, muscles located outside the joint also supply shock absorption and help keep the joint accurately aligned.

Since cartilage has no blood vessels, it depends on synovial fluid to supply nutrients. Compared with the bloodstream, synovial fluid is an inefficient method of supplying nutrients. For example, synovial fluid is unable to deliver repair enzymes which could be used to reproduce and to replace worn cartilage. Thus damaged cartilage cannot normally heal or replace itself by natural means.

Mind-made Arthritis

Extensive research into the function of the body's immune and stress responses have confirmed that the beliefs we hold in our minds are the largest single influence in causing arthritis.

41

When we hold beliefs that are predominently fear-based, we experience fear-based emotions like anger, hostility, guilt, anxiety, hopelessness, disappointment, resentment and depression. For example, believing that we should never forgive a slight or injustice almost invariably produces feelings of anger and resentment.

Whenever we experience such negative emotions, messenger molecules called "neuropeptides" swiftly relay our fear-based mood to receptors in our immune system cells. (The immune system is a complex organization of cells, bone marrow, antibodies and the thymus gland that defends the body against cancer and infections.)

Our immune system then mimics the way we feel. If we feel down and depressed, or angry, fearful or anxious, our immunity is suppressed and we become more vulnerable to cancer or infections.

In people with a genetic predisposition to RA, negative emotions may cause the immune system to act abnormally. Instead of defending the body against cancer and infections as it's supposed to, the immune system attacks joints in the body, creating inflammation and damaging cartilage with toxic secretions.

By contrast, positive beliefs and feelings are classified as love-based. When we perceive the world through a filter of love-based beliefs, we view it as friendly and nonthreatening, and we experience love, joy, compassion, optimism, hope, faith and cheerfulness.

As neuropeptide messengers relay these positive feelings to the immune system, it responds by increasing its ability to fight cancer and infections. The immune system also continues to function in a perfectly normal state of equilibrium. When this happens, RA and most other diseases rarely occur and we continue to enjoy high-level health. This comfortable, relaxed condition is known as the "relaxation response."

Stress: A Shapeless Destroyer of Body and Mind

The immune system isn't the only body mechanism to respond adversely to negative beliefs and emotions. The same fear-based beliefs and emotions that suppress and distort our immune response also trigger the body's fight-or-flight response. The fight-or-flight response is the body's arousal state, triggered by the mind whenever it perceives a situation as threatening or hostile. It is also known as the "stress response."

Stress occurs when we must adjust to a change or life event that we perceive as threatening or hostile to our comfort, safety, prestige or well-being. Modern life overflows with disturbing events and devastating social changes that can trigger stress. Layoffs, job loss, separation, divorce, retirement, bereavement or becoming a parent are all potential sources of stress.

A recent Louis Harris poll indicates that 33 percent of Americans experience severe stress for several days each week, while other millions are stressed out and exhausted by the pace and pressures of modern living. Nowadays, 83 percent of all visits to a doctor's office are due to symptoms arising from unresolved emotional stress. Stress impairs every aspect of the body-mind from the healing-regeneration system to physical and mental performance, sexual function and body weight.

Thus it's hardly surprising that many RA sufferers report that their symptoms first appeared during or shortly after a particularly stressful period. Millions of others have noticed that their flare-ups coincide with unusually stressful times. Frequently, the severity of the flare-up is in direct proportion to the amount of stress they experience.

The Anatomy of Stress

Anger, hostility, fear and resentment are among the principal fear-based emotions that trigger the fight-or-flight response, and all are considered prime causes of stress.

43

They work like this.

Whenever the mind perceives something as threatening or hostile, the brain's hypothalamus gland triggers the fight-or-flight response. This is a hair-trigger reaction that instantly readies the body to meet any threat to our survival. The adrenalin glands secrete stress hormones to speed up metabolism and the entire body-mind goes into a crisis mode.

Within a second, the muscles are energized and tensed for action. Heart and breathing rates speed up and breathing becomes rapid and shallow. Our blood vessels constrict and blood pressure soars. Digestion shuts down. The stomach produces a surplus of acid that irritates the stomach lining and frequently causes pain. To prevent bleeding in case of a wound, the body's blood-clotting mechanism is activated. The brain releases norepinephrine, a neurotransmitter that makes us hyperalert. And tissue cells release prostaglandins, hormonelike molecules that are intimately connected with inflammation and pain.

This response, a legacy from ancient times, prepares us to fight or flee from physical danger. Back in primitive times, our ancestors could defuse the fight-or-flight response by the physical act of fighting or by running away. This remedy still works. Ten minutes of vigorous exercise can totally dissipate the effects of the fight-or-flight response and relieve all the tension and discomfort that it causes.

Bottled-up Emotions May Spawn Arthritis

Such prompt relief is often impractical in modern life. It's difficult to fight or run away when we've just been bawled out by the boss in front of other employees. It's equally impractical on the freeway when someone cuts in front of us or in dozens of similar situations that trigger the fight-or-flight response.

44

The fight-or-flight response evolved to save us from physical danger. Obviously events like those just described pose zero physical danger. And responding to them with the fight-or-flight response is clearly an overreaction.

The problem is that the hypothalamus gland cannot distinguish whether a feeling of fear is triggered by a real and immediate danger, such as a charging bull, or whether it's the danger we imagine when we see an envelope in the mail from the IRS.

Whether the danger is real or imagined, the mind experiences fear. And our hypothalamus turns on the fight-or-flight response. In fact, the fight-or-flight response—or at least some of its mechanisms—can be turned on by almost any fear-based emotion. Whether it's fear, anger, hostility, anxiety, guilt or resentment, the hypothalamus triggers the fight-or-flight response.

Granted, a feeling of resentment won't turn on the same degree of alarm as a charging bull. But envy, depression, guilt or hopelessness are all fear-based emotions capable of turning on part of the fight-or-flight response.

Living Life on Overload

Urban life is filled with so many potentially stressful situations that many people live in a perpetual state of crisis with their fight-or-flight response continually simmering. These people are never truly relaxed and their life-support systems are in a continual state of emergency every hour of every day. The stress they experience is chronic.

However we turn on the fight-or-flight response, the result is much the same. At first, we experience an adrenalin rush that may make us feel empowered. But unless we can release the fight-or-flight response by exercise, or by a relaxation technique, we begin to feel muscular tension and a dull ache and discomfort all over the body. We may experience racing thoughts, a clenched jaw, sore joints and muscles, headaches, heart palpitations, depression and sweating, and we are left feeling exhausted and drained of energy.

It is these unpleasant and uncomfortable feelings that most people describe as "stress."

As science discovered that fear-based beliefs and stress are key components in many diseases, departments of behavioral medicine and stress-reduction clinics sprouted in most large hospitals and university medical centers. Some of these mind-body research centers have produced well-documented studies showing that when stress is reduced, the immune system is enhanced and its balance is restored. Nowadays, belief-reprogramming occupies a prominent place among topics taught by these centers.

Researchers have also discovered that we don't *have* to react with the fight-or-flight response to life events which are not life-threatening. We can easily learn to respond in less stressful ways that do not provoke arthritis or any other disorder. The techniques that have been developed for preventing and managing stress are described in several Arthritis Fighters later in this book.

Being Overweight Increases Arthritis Risk

Among other important discoveries is that millions of Americans, particularly women, use food as a tranquilizer to overcome the discomfort of stress. High-fat or sugar-laden foods will quickly relieve any discomfort in the stomach caused by the surfeit of acid released by the fight-or-flight response. But only at the cost of adding excess weight. Nowadays, one-fourth of Americans are at least 20 pounds overweight, and another fourth are 20 percent or more overweight, meaning they are obese.

Three-fourths of OA cases are due to being overweight. Researchers have also discovered that being overweight is a risk factor for RA as well. However, surplus weight is usually lost as RA progresses. But anyone who is 20 pounds or more overweight has a significantly higher risk of developing RA than a person of normal weight.

During the past decade, the average American added 8 pounds in weight. So it should come as no surprise that as Americans continue to gain weight, incidence of all forms of arthritis is increasing proportionally.

UNDERSTANDING RHEUMATOID ARTHRITIS

It remained for psychoneuroimmunologists to discover how the mind uses neuropeptides and neurohormones to communicate with the immune system—and with other mechanisms in our healing-regeneration system.

Take hormones first. Whenever a negative emotion turns on the fight-or-flight response, the adrenal glands release corticosteroid hormones, among which is cortisol, a powerful immunosuppressant. Chronic stress may elevate cortisol levels to the point where this hormone can create a serious imbalance in the immune system. Elevated cortisol levels are common in people with RA.

Corticosteroids contain the body's most powerful anti-inflammatory agent. Prolonged or chronic stress may eventually lead to a state of adrenal burnout that results in a deficiency of certain corticosteroids. Animal studies have demonstrated that the inability of the adrenals to release enough of these corticosteroids is often linked to the onset of inflammatory disorders such as RA.

Prostaglandins, other chemicals released by the fight-or-flight response, play a key role in regulating the inflammation and pain of RA.

Meanwhile, neuropeptide messengers travel through the nervous system, conveying information about our mood directly from the hypothalamus to white cells in the immune system—and to cells in other parts of the healing-regeneration system as well. Whether the mind is in a positive or negative mood, the cells in our body are swiftly informed. (Communication is also two-way. Body cells may also use neuropeptides to send messages to the brain.)

Your Beliefs Can Make You Sick or Make You Well

To make it clearer, *when we hold beliefs that are predominantly fear-based, we experience negative feelings that suppress and distort our immunity, making us more vulnerable to RA and many other diseases. The same negative feelings trigger the fight-or-flight response, which increases our risk for all stress-related diseases, particularly RA and OA.*

In contrast, when we view the world through a filter of love-based beliefs, we experience positive feelings that enhance our immunity and keep us in the relaxation response. This reduces our risk of ever getting RA and most other diseases.

By replacing fear-based beliefs with love-based beliefs, we can think ourselves well. Or by holding on to fear-based beliefs we can continue to suffer from RA and from a host of other stress-related conditions that can worsen arthritis.

Many physicians and researchers have observed that people with RA often seem to have a distinct personality profile. They tend to turn anger and other negative emotions inward rather than express their feelings. Many tend to be reserved and to avoid closeness, yet they are often dependent on others for support. RA sufferers tend to be perfectionists, to worry more than usual, to be nervous, restless, resentful, unforgiving, introverted and to be moody, high-strung and easily upset. Many also appear to adopt an outward facade of composure and self-assurance to mask a real deficiency of these traits. However, these are merely observations, not proven facts.

The Vigilant Warrior Cells of the Body's Immune System

The immune system is a complex organization of white blood cells, bone marrow, antibodies and the thymus gland that defends the body against invading viruses, bacteria and other sources of infectious disease. The immune system also destroys body cells that become cancerous and cells that are host to a virus. Though they are our own body cells, these cells are so changed by disease that immune system cells identify them as nonself and dangerous. In the remainder of this book, all nonself cells and viruses are known as "nonself substances."

Three types of immune system cells are involved in the immune response.

1. *T-cells* mature in the thymus gland.
T-helper cells patrol the bloodstream on a constant surveillance mission to detect any nonself substance. Actually, most nonself substances are first recognized by another type of immune cell called a macrophage (described below). The macrophage tears off a piece of the invader's outer surface, or antigen, and displays it for T-helpers to see. Then T-helpers set off a bodywide alarm and orchestrate the overall response of the entire immune system. T-helpers also stimulate B-cells (described below) to produce antibodies.

49

Natural killer (NK) cells are another type of T-cell which attacks and destroys tumors and other nonself substances during the immune response.

T-suppressor cells turn off the immune response after a nonself substance has been destroyed. T-suppressors work in tandem with T-helpers to maintain equilibrium in the immune system once the immune response is over. If they did not, the immune system would become increasingly aggressive, very possibly to the point where armies of white cells, mobilized to attack an invader, could roam through the bloodstream out of control and looking for other targets to attack.

2. B-Cells are so-called because they mature in the bone marrow and live there or in lymph glands. Once the immune response begins, B-cells manufacture and deploy antibodies designed to lock on to receptors in the nonself substance and disable it. When the target is destroyed, T-suppressor cells inhibit antibody production, and B-cells settle back into inactivity.

3. Macrophages are large white scavenger cells that patrol the bloodstream and are the first to recognize nonself substances and display their antigens for T-helpers to see. Macrophages are also able to engulf the remains of nonself substances after they have been disabled and destroyed.

The Body Fights Back

Macrophages and other immune cells identify a nonself substance by its antigen, a molecular recognition code carried in the protein walls of all cells and viruses. Both macrophages and T-helper cells recognize the antigen of every cell or virus they encounter and they identify it as self and friendly or as nonself and hostile.

Whenever a macrophage encounters a nonself substance, it tears off some antigens. Then, it swiftly displays these antigens and passes them to the nearest T-helper cell. The T-helper immediately sets off the immune response and the entire immune system swings into action.

NK cells migrate to the site through the bloodstream and attack and neutralize the nonself substances with their toxic enzymes.

Meanwhile, the T-helper cell alerts groups of B-cells in the vicinity and presents them with the invader's antigens. Immediately, large numbers of B-cells each divide into several plasma cells and begin to replicate antibodies specifically designed to match the sample antigens. Antibodies are Y-shaped, missilelike molecules that each lock on to two receptors on a nonself substance and paralyze it. When this happens, even the largest virus or cell can be subdued by other T-cells and macrophages. Macrophages then engulf and carry away the debris.

A different antibody is required for each type of virus or cell that invades the body. Certain B-cells are able to memorize the antibody pattern for every different nonself substance which has ever triggered the immune response during a person's life. Thanks to our B-memory cells, we become immune to diseases such as measles and mumps after a single attack. Nowadays, of course, vaccination uses the same memory mechanism to immunize a person against these and scores of similar infectious diseases.

During the immune response, increasing numbers of white cells are produced to help defend the body, and the body's white cell count rises.

When all nonself substances have been killed and destroyed, T-suppressor cells go into action and subdue the immune response.

When Our Immune System Goes Awry

In people with healthy emotions, the immune system functions splendidly to protect the body against cancer and infections. But when we experience stress and fear-based emotions, the brain despatches hormones and peptide messengers to every cell in the body.

When these messengers reach immune cells, the immune system translates their message into physical action. If we feel down and depressed or angry and stressed, activity of our T-helper cells is impaired and our immunocompetence is immediately suppressed. Nonself substances that are normally destroyed are then able to survive and multiply. This explains why a person with a high level of stress or depression is much more prone to develop cancer or to come down with an infectious disease.

In people who are genetically prone to RA, negative emotions or stress can throw the entire immune system off balance. Instead of suppressing the activity of T-helper cells, negative emotions or stress can distort the immune system so that the competence of T-suppressor cells is impaired. T-suppressor cells then fail to suppress the immune response, and the entire immune system begins to malfunction.

Renegade T-cells may attack T-suppressor cells while aberrant B-cells begin manufacturing autoantibodies. These are antibodies designed to lock on to receptors in the body's own cells and destroy them. The favorite target of autoantibody attack is collagen, a protein located in cartilage in the joints.

The Devastating Effects of Autoimmunity

This reaction is known as autoimmunity and diseases due to an immune imbalance are known as autoimmune diseases. Among them are RA, ankylosing spondylitis, lupus and scleroderma.

A well-balanced immune system shows a ratio of 1.8 T-helper cells to 1 T-suppressor cell. Higher or lower ratios indicate immune system malfunction. The ratio in a person with lupus is typically 1.5 to 1. By comparison, a deficiency of T-suppressor cells has been linked to RA. In people with some diseases that create a deficiency of T-suppressor cells, RA is 20 to 30 times more common than in the general public.

Few rheumatologists doubt that T-cell imbalance is responsible for most cases of RA. Tests show that when T-cells are removed from the bloodstream, symptoms of RA begin to disappear. Blood tests are also available that detect immune system abnormalities in people with RA.

RA occurs in two distinct stages. First, unresolved emotional stress causes an abnormality in the immune system known as autoimmunity. Second, autoimmunity swiftly expresses itself in a variety of symptoms known as autoimmune reactions. Among common autoimmune reactions are inflammation, pain, swelling, redness, heat and muscular stiffness in the afflicted joint; allergies; fatigue; poor digestion and appetite; loss of weight; and possibly a low-grade fever.

Disorders That Masquerade As Arthritis

Each of these, of course, is a common symptom of RA. But all too often, doctors and other health professionals regard these symptoms as the *cause* of RA, whereas, in reality, they are the *effect* of autoimmunity. Mainstream medicine often attempts to treat each of these symptoms with drugs. Practitioners of alternative medicine have also mistakenly identified autoimmune reactions, such as food allergies, as the cause of RA.

The cause of their confusion is that an aberrant immune system may trigger other autoimmune disorders that mimic the symptoms of RA but are not true arthritis. For example, an allergy to certain foods may produce pain and inflammation in a joint. But tests show that most people whose joint pain and inflammation is worsened by certain foods fail to show real symptoms of RA. For example, they fail to show joint deterioration and the presence of rheumatoid factor in the bloodstream. Nowadays, this dysfunction is known as "Allergic Arthritis" to distinguish it from RA or other authentic forms of arthritis. (How food allergies produce arthritislike symptoms is described in AF#12.)

Most types of allergies are actually autoimmune diseases. But they are not a form of arthritis. *However, the autoimmune disorders and reactions we're discussing in this chapter are those associated with genuine arthritis.*

Though it is possible to relieve some autoimmune reactions with drugs or a natural therapy, the underlying autoimmune process may continue to smoulder. Especially when a drug is used to alleviate one autoimmune reaction, another symptom may appear instead.

The Healing Power of Positive Beliefs

Natural therapies, such as our Arthritis Fighters, are often more successful. As you may recall from the preceding chapters, we can change the way we feel by changing the way we act. No action is involved in taking a drug. But to use a physical action-step such as heat and cold treatment or exercise, we must act. When we use our minds and muscles to act, we invoke inner healing powers such as the placebo and enabling effects while the brain releases pain-killing endorphins. By acting on the whole person, not merely on the joint we're trying to heal, natural therapies may boost our self-esteem to the point where our negative emotions are transformed into positive feelings.

Stress then disappears, balance is restored to the immune system and RA goes into remission. This remission continues for as long as we continue to use the natural therapy and to have faith and belief in its benefits. Or until we use stress management techniques to replace our negative beliefs with positive beliefs.

Inflammation Is the Most Common Autoimmune Reaction

Autoimmune reactions are the symptoms that tell us we may have RA. Inflammation is the most prominent and common symptom of RA.

If you have ever experienced pain, redness and swelling in any part of your body, it was probably due to inflammation, an important part of the immune response to an injury or infection. Inflammation is caused by secretions from several types of immune cells as they destroy viruses or bacteria or heal damaged tissue. In a normal immune system, once a nonself substance has been destroyed, T-suppressor cells turn off the inflammation process along with the rest of the immune response.

But once autoimmunity develops, the inflammation process continues unchecked. Since autoimmunity targets a joint, inflammation persists there. Usually, the target joint is in the toes, ankles, knees, hips, spine, shoulders, elbows, wrists or fingers. More than one joint may be attacked simultaneously, and it is common for the same joint to be affected on both sides of the body, a phenomenon called "symmetricality." Any inflamed joint may become swollen with fluid and be hot, tender and extremely painful.

Inflammation is a major symptom in all the more serious forms of autoimmune disease. Inflammation is provoked when substances such as complement and interferon are secreted by special CD4T cells and are aided and abetted by an influx of prostaglandins able to promote inflammation and pain. (Other types of prostaglandins can suppress inflammation.) Together, they start a chain reaction causing inflammation to multiply and spread.

How Autoimmunity Destroys Our Joints

In RA and other autoimmune diseases, autoantibodies, CD4T cells and prostaglandins all zero in on the inner lining, or synovial membrane, of the joint they are attacking. As the inflammation becomes chronic, the synovial membrane thickens, folds and develops fibers. Several types of immune cells are then able to locate in these nooks and crannies, all secreting chemicals that erode cartilage, bone, ligaments and the joint capsule itself. In severe cases of autoimmune disease, all eventually become misshapen and distorted, and the entire joint becomes grotesquely deformed. In severe cases of RA, a permanent joint deformity may develop in just one to two years.

Since RA is a systematic disease, inflammation may spread outside the joint. Rheumatoid nodules (lumps) may appear under the skin. RA may also inflame blood vessels, leading to a condition known as "vasculitis." One sign of vasculitis is the appearance of small brown spots or lines at the base of fingernails. People with RA may also bruise easily and develop blue or purple blotches under the skin. Others may develop neuritis or inflammation of one or more nerves. When nerves in the wrist are compressed, it is known as "carpal tunnel syndrome."

In more severe cases of RA, the heart may become inflamed, a condition known as "pericarditis." Inflammation can also spread to the eyes, nose, throat, lungs, vagina or kidneys, where it causes an annoying dryness.

The steps described so far in this chapter are those that lead to most cases of RA. A similar stress-caused autoimmune process is responsible for ankylosing spondylitis, lupus, scleroderma and other autoimmune diseases.

Rating the Severity of Rheumatoid Arthritis

Rheumatologists often rate the severity of RA by one of the four following categories.

1. Class 1 is the mildest form of RA. Some doctors refer to Class 1 as "monocyclic RA." Joint damage rarely occurs, and many patients make a complete and permanent recovery in under two years.

2. RA may smoulder much of the time but emerge periodically with a brief flare-up of symptoms.

3. More severe symptoms characterized by hot, painful and swollen joints and perhaps a low-grade fever. Four people out of ten with Class 3 or 4 RA find some difficulty in walking, sewing, typing, climbing stairs or opening doors, while some experience mild depression.

4. The most severe level, Class 4 RA may cause extensive damage during its early years, permanently crippling and disabling joints and severely limiting a person's quality of life. In rare cases, RA may become life-threatening. Some doctors refer to Class 4 as "malignant RA."

While complete proof is lacking, many doctors believe that aggressive treatment with powerful disease-remittive drugs is the only hope of minimizing the damage of Class 4 RA. These drugs are also known as "DMARDs" or "Disease-Modifying Anti-Rheumatic Drugs." They are very slow acting and must often be taken for months before any improvement appears. Adverse side effects are common, ranging from skin rash to mouth ulcers, nausea, immunosuppression, bone loss, vision impairment and possible damage to liver, lungs or kidneys.

Since it may take up to 20 years to thoroughly assess the benefits of this vigorous treatment, use of DMARDs is still considered controversial. Over the years, as RA symptoms gradually subside, milder-acting medications are substituted for these harsh and powerful drugs.

Autoimmunity Affects Women Differently

We know that stress hormones can trigger an immune system malfunction that leads to RA. But changes in hormone levels during pregnacy can also subdue the immune system in women and produce a remission from RA. One explanation is that the cells of a fetus are half self and half nonself and can be recognized by the mother's immune system as foreign. Hormones may emerge during pregnancy that subdue the immune system and prevent it from attacking a half-foreign fetus.

Whatever the explanation, most women with RA often feel better while pregnant. But after the birth, the disease may flare up again. In some women, the emotional stress of bearing a child has actually caused RA.

Although women have stronger and more active immune systems, they develop RA three times as often as men. Because women have a stronger antibody response than men, they have a higher resistance to infections. But their stronger ability to manufacture antibodies leads women to form autoantibodies more readily against collagen in their own joints.

Women given estrogen replacement therapy (ERT) may also see their RA symptoms improve. The same is true of women who take oral contraceptives. Both contain hormones which partially subdue the immune response.

In both men and women, however, an abnormal immune system is unable to seek out and destroy cancer cells and other invaders. Thus, having RA may lower your resistance to cancer and infections. Meanwhile, taking anti-inflammatory or other drugs could possibly increase risk of damage to the stomach, intestines, heart, lungs, kidneys or liver.

Other Conditions That Accelerate Autoimmunity

While stress is invariably the underlying cause of most autoimmune diseases, several convincing studies have suggested that other conditions may accelerate the disease process.

Aptosis is a process by which old, weak T-cells die and are replaced by young, active cells. When a mutation in a person's T-cells allows senescent cells to continue living, the T-cell population becomes defective and autoimmunity results. A severe infection may overload the immune system and create an imbalance. RA flare-ups often follow a severe cold or infection.

A Finnish study that followed 57,000 men for 30 years has indicated that male smokers have 8 times as much risk of developing RA as nonsmokers. Risk is also higher among male ex-smokers. No studies have been done on women. Heavy alcohol consumption also intensifies development of RA. In many cases, only gold salts can relieve RA symptoms in heavy drinkers.

Sleep deficiency has been clearly identified as a cause of immunosuppression, and insufficient sleep over a prolonged period is strongly suspected of disrupting the equilibrium of the immune system. A recent Louis Harris poll found one-third of Americans getting by on six hours or less of sleep per night. Another survey found that half of all men and women under 45 were sleep deficient.

A high-fat or high-calorie diet may also foster tremendous imbalances in the immune system. Back in the 1980s, Dr. Robert Good, a prominent immunologist, found that a diet high in calories speeds up shrinking of the thymus gland, the vital organ that processes new T-cells. A deficiency of T-cells may suppress immunity and seriously distort its balance. Also in the 1980s, Dr. Stuart Berger discovered that many overweight people had severe imbalances in their immune systems.

Rheumatoid Arthritis May Be Easier to Beat Than You Think

If you find this litany of symptoms and side effects depressing, take heart! A series of studies in Massachusetts showed that only 25 percent of people with RA are likely to experience more severe forms of the disease. Fewer than 5 percent end up in a wheelchair or are unable to care for themselves.

In 1987, for example, Dr. Lewis Kazis of Boston University Medical Center examined a group of 261 people who had suffered from RA for an average of nine years. All were tested to examine the extent of their symptoms and disabilities. When the same people were tested again five years later, no significant decrease was found in their manual dexterity nor in their ability to carry out daily physical activities.

Dr. Kazis concluded that over the years the health status of people with RA remained remarkably stable, with relatively few people experiencing a significant decline in health. And during the five-year period, the group did not show any appreciable change in levels of such negative emotions as anxiety or depression.

Another Massachusetts study turned up even more cheering news. A group of 118 people were examined and tested for severity of RA symptoms. All had unmistakable symptoms of RA. Between three and five years later, the same group was tested once again. At that time, only 28 percent reported having RA symptoms. Study authors concluded that:

- As a rule, 25 percent of people with RA are able to make a complete recovery.
- Fifty percent have symptoms that flare up part of the time but that generally stay in remission.
- The remaining 25 percent are likely to experience a Class 3 or 4 level of RA.

Study results indicated that 75 percent of RA sufferers will either have a total remission or experience symptoms of moderate intensity that wax and wane. If you are in this 75 percent, the Arthritis Fighter methods in this book can help you lead an almost normal life while boosting your chances of a permanent remission.

Most People Eventually Experience a Remission

Eventually, most people with RA experience a full or partial remission of symptoms. The remission may last for months or years or it may be permanent. And it can occur spontaneously regardless of any treatment or medication. However, many people have reported a remission after adopting a more positive mindset and attitude.

Up to 10 percent of people with RA experience a full or partial remission each year. As a rough guide, this means that people with Class 2 RA may anticipate a full or partial remission within 10 years after the disease first appears, people with Class 3 may expect a remission within 15 years, and people with Class 4 within 20 years.

A remission is defined as a great reduction, or a complete disappearance, of joint pain, inflammation, swelling, fatigue and other painful symptoms. Few remissions occur suddenly. Rather, each flare-up brings less pain and inflammation until the flare-ups subside entirely. A little joint pain and inflammation may linger, together with a few minutes of early morning stiffness. But these symptoms, too, should fade with time. Only irreparable damage to bone or joints remains as a reminder that RA once raged.

UNDERSTANDING OSTEOARTHRITIS

OA is a disease that degrades the cartilage in joints. It strikes most frequently in the knees, hips and spine of women over 50. And many people, including doctors, believe it is an inevitable part of the aging process.

But OA is *not* part of the aging process.

When a woman with OA in her right knee was told by her doctor that it was part of growing older, she asked: "Then is my left knee any younger?"

Although 68 percent of women over 65 show evidence of cartilage deterioration, OA is not a natural component of the aging process. Its most common cause is a combination of being overweight and sedentary living.

Weighing too much overloads our weight-bearing joints, creating excessive wear in the shock-absorbing cartilage. And failing to exercise causes our joints to stiffen up and lose flexibility. Simultaneously, the muscles around each joint—which also act as shock absorbers—atrophy from lack of use and no longer cushion the joint when we move or walk.

While OA affects twice as many women as men, it seldom appears in either sex before age 40. And even when cartilage deterioration occurs, it may be years before any symptoms appear. OA is most likely to occur in overweight women or in stocky, overweight men.

Osteoarthritis Can Strike People Under Forty

When it does hit men under 40, OA is usually due to an injury or a misalignment. For example, people who are bowlegged may be prone to OA symptoms. OA may also be caused by constant repetitive movement. Drivers of delivery vans who must open the doors many times each day often experience OA symptoms in their wrists and hands.

An injury or misalignment may also cause OA in younger women. But the most common type of OA to strike women under 40 is a mild form that causes painful bony nodules and neuritis pain in the joints of the fingers. These growths may make the fingers look unsightly, but the swelling is due to the bone growths, not to inflammation. Thus pain is often mild and movement is seldom impaired. After a year or two, symptoms usually fade away. Only the nodules remain.

As part of the big picture, however, injury, repetitive movement, misalignment and finger nodules are reponsible for only a small percentage of OA cases. An equally small percentage of OA may be due to genetically defective cartilage. If several family members who are blood relatives all have OA in both knees or in both elbows (or in other sym-

63

metrical joints), this may be a tipoff to a genetic cartilage defect.

In any case, OA symptoms due to an inherited cartilage defect are usually not experienced before age 45. And Arthritis Fighters, such as losing weight, may slow progression of genetically inherited OA for at least several years.

Osteoarthritis Appears Very Gradually

In most people, the first sign of OA is often a mild aching and soreness in the joint at the base of one of the thumbs or one of the big toes. After a while, early morning stiffness appears in a knee, hip or the spine. However, OA symptoms may also affect the shoulders, elbows, wrists and fingers. Usually, only one joint is affected.

As time goes on, stiffness may appear in the afflicted joint, especially after resting. Gradually, the joint becomes tender and painful to move. This leads most people to avoid moving that joint. Stiffness may then become chronic.

The less the joint is moved, the greater the discomfort when it is moved. An afflicted joint may crack or creak when moved, and OA in the knee often produces a gritty or grating sensation. OA in the hip may cause pain in the groin and inside the thigh. OA in the spine may lead to weakness and numbness in legs, shoulders, arms, neck and back, or it may even cause headaches, earache or a sore throat.

But OA is not systematic. Pain and damage are usually confined to the afflicted joint. Most people with OA experience more stiffness than inflammation. Pain is usually moderate and the disease is rarely crippling. However, severe OA in the knees or hips can cause a person to limp or shuffle and may eventually lead to disability. Curiously, severe joint damage may cause only mild pain while mild joint damage may cause severe pain.

Overweight and Inactivity Cause Most Osteoarthritis

Evidence identifying overweight and sedentary living as the root cause of OA is well documented. According to a long-term study of graduates from John Hopkins School of Medicine (reported in the *University of California Wellness Letter*, February 1995), young men in their twenties who are 20 pounds or more overweight almost double their risk of developing OA in the knees and hip later in life.

More evidence comes from a 1992 review of 1,416 people by the Framingham Heart Study. The authors discovered that exercise did *not* increase risk of OA in the knee. In fact, OA is seldom seen in any active person who stays fit and trim. The Framingham Study also discovered that overweight and older women could halve their risk of getting OA of the knee by losing 11 pounds over a ten-year period. The same reduced risk is believed to apply to men also.

Older athletes also show much less OA than sedentary people. A 1985 study at the Florida Veterans Administration Medical Center in Gainesville found that runners in their 50s and 60s face far less risk of OA or knee degeneration than sedentary people of the same age. Researchers found that joints, cartilage and bones in the runners were much stronger than those in sedentary people in their 50s and 60s.

OA begins when the stress of bearing excessive weight softens and frays the cartilage that pads the ends of bones in a joint. In a joint afflicted with OA, the cartilage pads become pitted and worn. The cartilage hardens and loses its elasticity and ability to absorb shock. When this happens, the cartilage gradually wears thin until the underlying bone is exposed. Thick bone spurs called "osteophytes" grow on the exposed bone and cysts filled with fluid may form in the joint.

As the remaining cartilage becomes brittle, loose pieces

break off and drift in between the joint surfaces, causing sharp pain. Unless treated, the entire joint structure may eventually disintegrate, leaving the joint deformed and misshapen.

UNDERSTANDING GOUT

Ten years of discussing business deals over cocktails, rich lunches and dinners left 45-year-old James overweight and out-of-shape. Then, without warning, James was jolted awake in the middle of the night with a searing, throbbing pain in his right big toe.

James was horrified when he looked at his toe. It was shiny, swollen and reddish-purple in color, and it was so exquisitely tender that James could not even bear to touch it.

It was two days before the pain and inflammation had subsided sufficiently to allow James to visit a doctor. The doctor immediately diagnosed James's problem as gout.

James swiftly learned that gout begins when men respond to the stresses of life by indulgent eating and sedentary living. Approximately 2 million Americans have gout and 95 percent are overweight, middle-aged men who never exercise.

"Gout is caused by rich foods and alcohol that leave an excess of uric acid in the bloodstream," the doctor said. "Eventually, the acid sinks to the lowest extremity of the body and deposits sharp-pointed monosodium urate crystals in the synovial fluid surrounding the joint of the big toe. These needle-sharp crystals are then attacked by large immune-system cells called "macrophages." But the cells can't destroy the crystals. So, instead, the macrophages release toxic chemicals that intensify the pain and inflammation to the point where it's almost unbearable."

The doctor explained that we don't hear much about gout these days because it is easily controlled by oral medications that slow the rate at which the body produces uric acid.

"But all the drugs do is to mask symptoms," the doctor went on, "and they can make you feel drowsy or upset your stomach. Most people with gout are willing to tolerate these side effects because the drugs allow them to go on eating and drinking the same things that caused their gout in the first place. But this high-fat diet and sedentary lifestyle puts them at risk for heart disease, stroke, cancer, diabetes and a host of other life-threatening diseases."

Most Gout Attacks Can Be Eliminated Naturally

Then the doctor told James that three-fourths of all gout cases can be almost totally eliminated without drugs by switching to a healthier diet and by losing weight and exercising.

The choice was up to James. He could either take a drug for life and continue with his health-destroying lifestyle and diet. Or he could adopt a sane and stress-free lifestyle.

"I'd like to think it over for a couple of days," he told the doctor.

James immediately headed for the public library and began reading everything he could find on gout. There, he swiftly learned that gout is the most painful of all forms of arthritis.

It begins with a diet high in such foods as organ meats, oily fish, chocolate, coffee, beer and wine. Foods like these have a high content of certain proteins known as "purines" and "xanthines." Both break down into uric acid, which is normally filtered out and excreted by the kidneys. But in a person who is overweight and sedentary, the kidneys are often so sluggish that they cannot handle the excessive supply of uric acid. Instead, uric acid spills into the bloodstream.

Gravity carries it to the lowest level of the body—the big toe—where it crystallizes in the joint lining. Any movement then drives the needle-like crystals into the synovium, producing severe irritation and inflammation and triggering macrophage attacks.

James read that the initial attack can be quite mild. But if left untreated, or if the sufferer continues to indulge in rich foods and alcohol, attacks become more frequent and severe. Many sufferers say that gout pain is like being constantly pounded on the big toe with a hammer. Eventually, gout can spread to other joints, causing stiffness and possible damage to the bone. After several years, the excess of uric acid may form gravel or stones in the kidneys or lead to kidney disease.

A tendency to gout may be inherited, but the disease itself can often be avoided by staying slender, eating healthfully and exercising daily. Psoriasis or leukemia may also produce symptoms of gout. And gout may appear as an adverse side effect of medications such as diuretics or antihypertensive drugs.

Extinguishing Gout Pain with Wise Health Choices

James told me the story of his gout when I sat next to him at lunch during a health convention. The lunch was strictly vegetarian, a far cry from the high-protein foods of animal origin that had caused James's gout attack.

It was learning all about gout, he told me, that transformed his relationship to stress and health.

"As I learned how gout functions, I realized I was doing and eating everything that made gout worse," he said. "A drug might save me from the pain of gout, but if I continued my gout-provoking lifestyle, I'd be at risk for the even greater pain of a heart attack or cancer."

So for the first time in his life, James began making wise health choices.

Two days after seeing his doctor, James began a program of exercise, stress management and weight reduction under medical supervision. That was almost five years ago. When I met him, James was slender, relaxed and totally free of any stiffness or pain.

The program he followed is almost identical to that in Arthritis Fighter #13.

Learning the Facts Helps You Take Control of Your Arthritis

If you have absorbed this chapter so far, you probably know as much about the genesis of arthritis as many doctors. In fact, many health professionals fail to recognize that arthritis is the body's reaction to deep-rooted stress. Nor do the majority of physicians realize that the balance of our immune system is under our direct, personal control. The Arthritis Fighters in this book allow us to personally intervene at every level in the arthritis process.

If you have arthritis, increasing your knowledge is the first step in gaining power over your disease. To become a medically educated layperson, I recommend reading this book right through to the end. Each chapter and Arthritis Fighter contains important new information that will expand your knowledge of arthritic disease.

I'm sure you are already aware that ignoring the early warning signs of arthritis may lead to irreparable damage later. Incredibly, however, statistics show that the average person does not seek medical diagnosis until four-and-a-half years after arthritis symptoms first appear.

To help you avoid this pitfall, the next chapter introduces the various types of health professionals who diagnose and treat arthritis. And it guides you through the maze of treatment options currently available.

CHAPTER FOUR

The Pros and Cons of Medical Treatment— and When to Seek Help

If you think you have arthritis, at what point should you see a doctor? And which type of doctor should you see? These are the classic warning signs of arthritis:

- Early morning stiffness before you get out of bed every day, which may take up to 30 minutes to loosen up.
- Inability to move a joint properly through its full range of motion.
- Swelling, redness and warmth in a joint.

- Tenderness or pain in a joint, especially if it is tender to the touch or hurts when squeezed.
- If any of the above symptoms persist for two weeks or longer, you should see a doctor. If these symptoms are also associated with unexplained fatigue, fever, weight loss or weakness, you should see a doctor promptly.

When a joint is red, warm and swollen, but ibuprofen or aspirin alleviates the pain until the effects wear off, that could indicate an infection that might cause serious cartilage damage in just one or two weeks. So see a doctor promptly.

You should also see a doctor if joint pain is compromising your daily activities or interfering with sleep, or if joint symptoms are symmetrical, that is, occurring in the same joint on both sides of the body.

Meanwhile, avoid doing any impact exercise of a painful joint until it has been examined by a doctor.

Which Type of Doctor Should You See?

Since you may need a referral before you can see a specialist, the best place to start is with a primary physician such as a *general practitioner, family doctor* or *internist.* While none is specially trained in arthritis, internists do receive three additional years of graduate training after completing medical school. Thus internists may be more familiar with the symptoms of RA than other primary care physicians, and they may be quicker to spot an infection that might be mimicking the symptoms of RA.

At times, I've heard complaints that all three types of primary care physicians have been slow to recognize RA symptoms and to treat Class 4 RA aggressively. If your symptoms resemble those of severe RA, try to have your primary care physician refer you to a rheumatologist for a clear diagnosis.

Rheumatologists are primarily internists who have received two additional years of graduate training in arthritis and other diseases of joints, bones and connective tissue. Their skill at making an accurate diagnosis has never been questioned, but they do tend to medicalize everything and to use drugs extensively. The big problem is that only a few thousand exist and only two-thirds of those may actually be board-certified in rheumatology. Nonboard-certified rheumatologists are usually experienced physicians who specialize in arthritis. To locate a board-certified rheumatologist, contact your local chapter of the Arthritis Foundation (see Appendix), a university hospital or county medical society, or look in the Yellow Pages under Arthritis or Rheumatology. If you have moderate-to-severe RA, a rheumatologist is your best bet.

Other Physicians Who Specialize in Arthritis

If you have a knee pain or OA, or believe you may require joint surgery, consider an orthopedist. *Orthopedists* are surgeons who receive five years of graduate training in diseases of the joints and bones. They perform repairs and reconstructive surgery on deformed and damaged joints, cartilage, tendons, ligaments and muscles. Orthopedists are also experienced in treating OA that does not require surgery. If you need surgery for any damaged joint, you will need an orthopedist. But since not all surgery is successful, you should obtain a second opinion from a rheumatologist, if possible, before agreeing to surgery.

For OA or for any kind of physical therapy or rehabilitation, a *physiatrist* (fizz-eye-a-trist) would be a sound choice. Physiatrists are M.D.s who have received four years of graduate training in physical rehabilitation. They frequently prescribe exercise to strengthen muscles and are experts in the use of heat and cold, water therapy, ultrasound and immobilizing joints with splints to permit rest. They prefer natural methods to drugs and are often knowledgeable about nutrition. Most practice only in large city hospitals or medical centers.

For a medical doctor who is more open to natural therapies, an osteopathic physician may be your best bet. A doctor of osteopathy (D.O.) is a medical doctor with additional training in bone, muscle and joint problems. Although fully qualified to prescribe drugs and perform surgery, D.O.s often prefer to employ more natural methods like using the hands or palpitations for diagnosis. They're often experts in using exercise, heat and cold therapy, spinal manipulation and nutrition. Many practice in smaller cities and a referral may not be necessary.

The Medical Exam

Whichever type of doctor you see, he or she will begin by finding out about your symptoms and making a careful history. If he or she suspects RA, your doctor will conduct a physical exam to look for skin rashes, inflammation, stiffness and immobility in joints and for signs of infection, fever, weakness or weight loss. Finally, you'll be given a series of tests that may include a complete blood count and tests for rheumatoid factor and sedimentation rate.

Rheumatoid factor is an antibody in the blood that inhibits inflammation. A high rheumatoid factor count indicates a high level of inflammation and a high probability that RA exists. Approximately two-thirds of people with RA have rheumatoid factor in their blood, but a high rheumatoid factor level may also be due to cancer, lupus, an infection or tubercolosis. At least 5 percent of healthy people also have rheumatoid factor in their bloodstream yet have no symptoms of RA. Thus a positive rheumatoid factor test does not actually confirm the existence of RA. It merely indicates an increased probability.

A sedimentation rate test measures the speed at which red blood cells settle to the bottom of a test tube. The faster the cells clump together and sink, the more inflammation a person has. While most people with RA have a rapid sedimentation rate, this test confirms only the extent of a person's inflammation. Cancer or an infection may also speed up the sedimentation rate. So while a high sedimentation rate also indicates a high probability of RA, it does not verify the existence of the disease.

Because no single test can clearly diagnose RA, your doctor is likely to use a variety of tests and to pool their results. For instance, a reduced red blood cell count is another indication of RA, while a high white cell count often indicates an infection. Your doctor may also test your urine or make a culture to identify an infection. If gout is suspected, a sample of synovial fluid may be withdrawn from an afflicted joint by needle aspiration and analyzed immediately in your doctor's office. If necessary, a sample of joint tissue may also be extracted through a hollow-core needle for analysis in the lab.

When results from the tests, the physical exam and your history are assessed together, most doctors can make a fairly accurate diagnosis. However, it may take two or three visits to your doctor and a variety of tests before a clear diagnosis is possible. That's because your doctor may want to ensure that your symptoms are not being caused by one of several common disorders that mimic arthritis.

For example, arthritislike symptoms *could* be due to a torn cartilage, a bone fracture, bursitis or tendinitis, a muscle or ligament injury, or to fibromyalgia, Lyme Disease or an infection. Until these possibilities have been ruled out, a clear diagnosis is often impossible.

Are You Genetically Prone to Rheumatoid Arthritis?

Eventually, new and better diagnostic tests may become available. For example, genetic markers usually exist on the surfaces of B-cells in people with RA and other autoimmune diseases. Each marker is specific to a certain disease. Over 60 percent of people with RA have the antigen HLA-DR4, but this marker occurs in only 27 percent of people free of RA. Most people with lupus carry the marker HLA-B8, and those with ankylosing spondylitis carry the marker HLA-B27. In fact, the ankylosing spondylitis marker occurs in 95 percent of all whites and 50 percent of blacks who have the disease.

While having a genetic marker indicates a strong predisposition to one or other forms of autoimmune disease, it does not guarantee you will actually get the disease. Fewer than 20 percent of people with the ankylosing spondylitis marker are actually hit by the disease. Nonetheless, if one of your parents or a sibling had RA, you are 4 times as likely to develop it as the average person.

Even if you have a genetic susceptibility to an autoimmune disease, you can dramatically cut your risk of ever getting it by incorporating some or all of our Arthritis Fighters into your lifestyle. For example, only 66 percent of identical twins both develop RA. One third don't. Our Arthritis Fighters offer a splendid way to protect yourself from arthritis by preventing it from ever developing.

Early Warning Signs of Arthritis

If one or more close relatives has developed arthritis, you can test yourself for early warning signs of OA or RA. Each test below should reveal the possible early presence of arthritis long before the usual pain and symptoms occur. If you can hold each position without joint pain for 5 full seconds, you should be free of arthritis. If joint pain occurs, it may indicate the possible onset of arthritis in the painful joint.

Caution: These tests do not indicate gout. Do not continue to bend or put pressure on any joint if obvious pain occurs. And do not use these tests on any joint which is stiff, inflamed or has been injured, nor if you have osteoporosis. These are tests, not exercises for improving range of motion.

Test 1. Place your hands behind your back with the flat of your hands on the small of the back or upper buttocks. Move your elbows back as far as you can. Any discomfort in spine, neck, shoulders or elbows may be a harbinger of arthritis in these joints.

Test 2. Place both hands on top of your head with the elbows pushed well back. Discomfort in shoulders or elbows may indicate nascent arthritis.

Test 3. Place both hands behind your back and slide your hands up your spine as far as you can. Any discomfort in neck, spine, shoulders, elbows, wrists or hands may indicate possible arthritis.

Test 4. Sit in a straight-backed chair with feet flat on the floor. Keep your back straight against the back of the chair. Then lean forward and down. Keep your arms outside your knees and touch your toes. Any discomfort in spine, knees, ankles, shoulders, elbows or hands could be a predictor of arthritis in these joints.

Test 5. Place both hands behind your neck with elbows extended sideways. Push your elbows back as far as you can. Any discomfort in neck, shoulders, elbows or hands could be a tip-off of approaching arthritis.

Test 6. Press the palms of both hands together in front of your face with elbows extended sideways. Any discomfort in shoulders, elbows or hands could reveal early arthritis.

What Your Hands Can Tell You

The following early warning signs of developing arthritis may also occur in the hands:

- A warm, inflamed swelling of the upper and middle joints of fingers may indicate early onset of RA. (The upper joint is the knuckle where the finger joins the hand.)
- A bony, hard swelling of the middle and lower (next to the nail) joints may be an early sign of OA.
- Small white deposits under the skin and next to any finger joint may indicate gout.
- Tiny dark red hemorrhages under the fingernails could be an early sign of lupus.
- If the skin on hands and fingers appears to be drawn tight so that wrinkles disappear, it could be an early sign of scleroderma.
- Should a fingernail become thick and soft to the touch, and also change color to an opaque white, it could warn of Reiter's Syndrome, a form of arthritis that sometimes occurs in young men.

• A hard, bony swelling of the upper knuckles—known as Hemochromatic Arthritis—could be caused by too much iron in the diet.

These early warning signs merely indicate that arthritis *may* be developing; they are not unmistakable signals that you have the disease. They're simply intended to alert you to the possibility of approaching arthritis, not to turn you into a hypochondriac or send you running to a doctor. Normally, you need not see a doctor until more definite symptoms, such as those discussed at the beginning of this chapter, have appeared.

The real value of these early warning signs is to give you a head start in preventing arthritis from ever occurring. By adopting the specific Arthritis Fighters recommended in Chapter 5 for OA, RA or gout, and making them a permanent part of your lifestyle, you can probably prevent arthritis from ever developing.

What to Expect from Medical Treatment

As this was written, medical science had no cure for OA or RA. Instead, doctors focused on three aims:

• To relieve pain, inflammation and other symptoms.
• To retard progress of the disease and to prevent further joint damage.
• To restore movement and flexibility to afflicted joints.

To achieve this, doctors often prescribe several therapies to be used together. Typically, these would be drugs, heat and cold treatment, physical therapy, exercise and psychological counseling. Doctors may also prescribe splints to protect a painful joint from stress and to hold it in a comfortable position during sleep.

Whether you have OA, RA or gout, physicians usually begin by prescribing first line drugs such as NSAIDs (aspirin or ibuprofin) to relieve pain and reduce inflammation. To effectively relieve chronic pain, however, as many as 16 aspirin tablets must be taken each day. A dosage this high often leads to disturbing side effects such as intestinal bleeding or a ringing in the ears.

Medical Treatment for Osteoarthritis

For OA, your doctor may begin by X-raying the joint for possible damage or misalignment. And if a weight-bearing joint is involved, and you are overweight, a weight-loss program will be recommended. Drugs, other than analgesics, are seldom prescribed.

Since cartilage has poor blood supply, it will not normally heal or restore itself naturally. For this reason, most treatment for OA is based on weight loss and physical rehabilitation. An important step in recovery nowadays consists of strengthening the muscles of an afflicted joint. Strong muscles not only promote joint flexibility, but they provide the extra shock absorption that allows a damaged joint to be used actively and without pain once again.

Nowhere is this more apparent than in knee joints. Because it depends on soft tissue for stability, the knee is an easily damaged joint. Pads of tough, slippery cartilage called "menisci," which cushion the lower surface of the joint, are especially susceptible to being torn or damaged.

Like all cartilage, the menisci receive nutrients from synovial fluid which is secreted only in response to movement. While walking, waste products are squeezed out of the menisci as weight is placed on the knee during the power step.

Fresh nutrients are then absorbed as weight is removed from the knee during the recovery step. Regular exercise is an absolute requirement to create this nutrient exchange which is essential for healthy knees. Thus it's not surprising that most knee damage occurs in sedentary people. Menisci damage in active people is usually caused by a sports injury.

Any pain in the lower knee joint usually involves the menisci. Often, it is caused when tiny fragments of frayed cartilage break off and enter the joint. After a few days, the fragment wears away and the pain disappears—until another fragment breaks off. While this is not true OA, it *is* a common form of arthritis. And unless treated, it will continue to wear away cartilage until full-blown OA appears.

Chondromalacia is another equally common type of knee pain. Chondromalacia begins when cartilage wears away on the inside of the kneecap (patella). Frequently, the cause is weak hamstring or quad muscles in the thigh. When one set of these muscles is stronger than the other, they distort the track of the patella over the thigh bone, wearing away cartilage in the process.

Both chondromalacia and menisci damage are commonly due to weakness in the hamstring or quad muscles, much of it due to sedentary living. As a first step to recovery, most knowledgeable doctors nowadays recommend strengthening these muscles with strength-building exercises based on using a knee exercise machine in a gym.

A Natural Therapy Restores a Damaged Knee to "Like-New" Condition

I can personally confirm the powerful benefits of strength-building exercises. In 1981, when I lived in Colorado, I tore a meniscus in a skiing accident. An orthopedist recommended

81

leg extension exercises using weights. At that time, I did not have access to a knee exercise machine and I had to use weights tied to a boot. This crude arrangement wasn't very effective. Eventually, the orthopedist operated on my knee using a new procedure called "arthroscopy."

Back then, little was known about proper rehabilitation. My knee did not recover fully and I was unable to exercise by cross-country skiing. During the Colorado winter, this was about the only aerobic exercise possible outdoors. After a year with little improvement, I moved to South Texas where I could bicycle year round. That helped. But what helped even more was that in Texas, the local gym had a knee exercise machine.

The quad muscles I used in bicycling were strong. But the opposing hamstrings weren't. At least, not until I'd worked out on the knee machine for several weeks.

Suddenly, I found I could walk ten or twelve miles without pain. Next summer, I returned to Colorado and hiked to the top of several of the state's highest peaks. Since then, I've hiked and bicycled through the Alps, the Andes and the Himalayas without any problems. Only when I'm away from home for an extended period, and unable to exercise on the knee machine, does any hint of knee pain ever return.

When Arthroscopy May Help

When all else fails, an orthopedist may suggest an arthroscopy operation. At most hospitals, this is an out-patient procedure during which thin tubes are inserted into the knee under general or local anasthesia. Tiny surgical tools are slid through the tubes and used to smooth damaged cartilage inside the knee. Results are usually successful, but don't expect your knee to be quite as good as new. As I discovered, however, when arthroscopic surgery is combined with muscle strengthening, I could do almost everything I used to do, short of high-impact activities like running.

New developments promise even better results for arthroscopy. In 1995, researchers at the University of Utah School of Medicine found that when arthroscopy was used merely to irrigate and wash all stray fragments out of the joint, results were almost comparable with surgery. And unlike surgery patients, who must rehabilitate the knee for weeks after the operation, wash-out patients regain full use of the knee in just a day or two.

Another promising arthroscopy procedure involves cell transplants. First, small pieces of knee cartilage are removed from an undamaged area. They are then separated and regrown in a test tube for several weeks. Finally, the new cells are injected back into the knee. Though still experimental at this time, the new cartilage that results appears to cushion joints almost as well as the original. The procedure seems to work best on isolated areas of damaged cartilage. It cannot yet be used to repair an entire joint or to reverse OA.

Today, orthopedists can repair almost any joint with a metal or plastic replacement. Or they can reconstruct a joint deformed by RA so that it functions effectively once more. Thus far, hip replacements have proven most successful. Artificial joints elsewhere may still loosen after many years. Or they may become infected and have to be replaced again.

While estrogen replacement therapy (ERT) isn't a medication for OA, several surveys report that women on ERT have a 30 percent lower risk of developing OA than other women. And among women who have OA, those taking estrogen reported 50 percent less pain and disability. ERT is believed to inhibit loss of both cartilage and bone. Don't expect your doctor to prescribe ERT merely to prevent OA. But if you are already taking estrogen, your risk of developing OA should be well below average.

Medical Treatment for Gout

If you have gout symptoms, your doctor should first make sure they are not due to pseudo-gout. This step is necessary because goutlike symptoms are often associated with psoriasis, leukemia or septic arthritis, or they could be triggered by a diuretic medication.

Gout often responds well to an all-natural, whole-person approach based on weight reduction; a low-fat, plant-based diet; a gradually increasing program of daily exercise; and the elimination of alcohol. But for those unwilling to make these lifestyle changes—and that includes most of America's 2 million gout sufferers—doctors generally prescribe one or other of two widely used anti-gout medications. By retarding the rate at which the body produces uric acid, these medications protect men with gout from having to give up their gout-producing lifestyle.

Each medication is taken orally and, once begun, must be continued for life. The reason is that, if not treated, gout can spread to other joints and may eventually damage and disable the body. Untreated gout may also lead to diabetes, heart disease or hypertension. However, these drugs are not without such adverse side effects as drowsiness or stomach upset.

Once drug treatment is begun, the only escape is to begin a program of exercise, weight loss, dietary improvement and abstinance from alcohol under medical supervision. For a whole-person program to overcome gout without drugs, see AF#13.

Medical Treatment for Rheumatoid Arthritis

Medical treatment for RA depends on the severity of symptoms. In fact, very mild cases of what appears to be Class 1 RA may cause only minor discomfort, while a sedimentation rate test fails to find any inflammation. Instead of treating these mild symptoms, your doctor may wait until a more positive diagnosis of RA becomes possible.

In about 50 percent of very mild RA cases, disease symptoms gradually disappear. But in other cases, pain and inflammation may flare up and keep returning until they become chronic.

Should RA progress to Class 3 or 4 levels, most doctors currently believe that only swift and aggressive drug treatment can prevent serious damage to cartilage and bone. Early in the onset of Class 4 RA, a patient feels sore, stiff, tired and aches all over. Joints swell and stiffen, become hot and tender, and a variety of skin disorders may appear. Hopefully, if this happens, you'll be under the care of a rheumatologist.

The standard practice currently used is to begin treatment with DMARDs, powerful second line antirheumatic drugs that may include antimalarial and immunosuppressive medications and gold salts. To retard severe RA and protect your joints, you may have to take these, or similar drugs, for several years.

I've already stated that most of these drugs have adverse and unpleasant side effects. For that reason, as soon as symptoms diminish, your doctor will replace them with less potent drugs. But that can take several years.

Eventually, drugs that are less harsh may be developed. As this book goes to press, some doctors are experimenting with a new antibiotic believed to break down the enzyme responsible for destroying cartilage in RA. Other doctors are experimenting with lower dose combinations of second line drugs that result in lessened side effects.

Every Drug Is a Double-Edged Sword

However, as this was written, so many people had experienced adverse side effects from almost every type of arthritis drug that thousands of arthritis sufferers were turning to natural, nonpharmaceutical remedies. And no wonder! The side effects of just one commonly prescribed drug for RA included a distinct possibility of lung disease, weight loss, fatigue, loss of appetite, reduced immunity and depression, as well as hair loss or sores on the inside of the mouth or skin.

Certainly, not every patient experiences side effects quite this severe. But many arthritis drugs have fallen into disrepute because of their excessive and intolerable side effects. Moreover, several commonly prescribed second line drugs work for fewer than 50 percent of patients. While most of these drugs are *believed* to slow the progress of RA, little scientific proof exists to substantiate that hypothesis.

Nowadays, new arthritis drugs are constantly being developed. Many are introduced with great fanfare. But after a few months, the majority prove too unpleasant to take or are less effective than advertised. One rheumatologist advises never taking a new drug until at least a million people have taken it first.

Other rheumatologists are using drugs for off-label purposes, that is, for diseases other than those that the drug was developed for. In many cases, long-term effects have not been studied. For example, immunosuppressive drugs are widely used to weaken immune cells responsible for autoimmunity. Yet these drugs significantly increase the risk of cancer or infections, and patients' blood must be monitored regularly for formation of new blood cells. Otherwise, these drugs can cause liver damage or life-threatening bone marrow suppression.

Penicillin-type drugs are another class of off-label medication prescribed for RA. Many people are unable to tolerate these drugs, and unless carefully monitored, they may cause kidney damage, muscle weakness or bone marrow suppression.

A Common Drug That Is Frequently Overused

Low cost aspirin ranks as one of the most effective nonnarcotic remedies for pain, fever and inflammation. Yet in the quantities required to be effective in relieving RA, a significant number of patients experience undesirable side effects.

Furthermore, both aspirin and other NSAIDs have been suspected of accelerating cartilage degeneration and destruction. The suspicion focuses on the ability of NSAIDs to inhibit synthesis of a strong collagen matrix that worsens OA at a faster-than-normal pace. Aspirin reduces inflammation through a similar process by blocking production of prostoleukotrienes, a prostaglandin that protects the stomach lining. When this happens, which is often, aspirin causes gastrointestinal irritation and bleeding.

To some extent, that can be prevented by taking coated aspirin (which takes longer to work). Or you can take a second drug to prevent stomach irritation, but this, too, has side effects, and up to 12 percent of patients have reported diarrhea and abdominal pain. An aspirin substitute like acetaminophen has fewer side effects but fails to reduce inflammation (nonetheless, it does reduce the pain of OA).

Pharmaceutical Overkill

Some RA patients I interviewed said they had tried as many as 20 different drugs, none of which was really effective. Almost all had experienced a high level of drug toxicity. Small women are especially vulnerable to a high level of toxicity from RA drugs. That's because most drugs come in standard-sized, fixed-dosage pills designed for a person of average height and weight. Older people, too, are unable to excrete drug toxicity as rapidly as younger people. That makes it difficult for doctors to reduce the dosage for smaller or older people.

Instead, doctors must monitor these patients by taking urine and blood tests every two months to check for damage to kidney or liver. One cancer drug commonly used in treating RA is so toxic to body cells that it has caused nausea and vomiting in one person in five and requires a monthly liver profile blood test to check for liver damage.

Most of us have probably experienced an itching skin rash after taking a powerful drug. While it may seem just a minor irritation, in reality an itching rash indicates that the drug is toxic to the human body and may cause serious damage if use is continued.

All this has led some doctors to suggest that NSAIDs and other arthritis drugs are being overused. Kidney damage is a common result of drug overuse. These and other problems connected with arthritis drugs—not to mention the expense—have caused millions of people to wonder whether it is all worthwhile.

Drugs Are No Panacea

The disturbing part about focusing on drugs is that roughly one-third of any improvement is due to the placebo effect—an integral part of the body-mind's natural healing-regeneration system. Also, drugs are often given credit when a remission occurs naturally or as the result of an alternative therapy. Moreover, by relying on drugs, doctors overlook the fact that emotional stress is the underlying cause of most forms of arthritis. In many cases, a stress management or exercise program, or both, might achieve far better results without the side effects of drugs.

Yet the medical profession is not entirely to blame. Most Americans prefer to pop a pill than to actively use their minds and muscles to beat arthritis naturally. Besides, it takes only five minutes to write a prescription versus an hour to explain how to use a series of natural techniques.

This widespread public apathy discourages many doctors from recommending natural therapies. Although virtually the entire medical community agrees that exercise is the one best therapy to relieve stiffness in joints, fewer than 25 percent of patients stay with an exercise routine—even when it clearly helps.

Furthermore, doctors are under tremendous pressure from pharmaceutical salespeople to prescribe drugs. So the medical profession isn't entirely at fault. The sad part is that almost everyone is swept into the drug trap —including people who *are* willing to use natural therapies.

How to Liberate Yourself from the Drug Trap

If your arthritis medication obviously isn't working . . . or the side effects are unbearable . . . or if an alternative therapy you are using seems to help more than your medication, see your doctor.

You *must* have your doctor's permission to change to a different medication, reduce the dosage or stop it altogether. If you have an autoimmune disease, your doctor may have a good reason for continuing with your present medication. Otherwise, you might consider asking him or her to switch to a more gentle medication, reduce the dosage or cut it out entirely. *Clearly, however, you must not stop taking any medication without your doctor's approval.*

While seeing your doctor, be sure to ask for his or her

permssion before you use any or all of the Arthritis Fighter techniques in this book. No one with arthritis, or any other disease or dysfunction, should commence an exercise program, change his or her diet or practice any psychological technique without a physician's approval.

If you have arthritis symptoms, a medical diagnosis is essential. And some medical treatments are obviously life-saving. But as any doctor can tell you, if you already have OA, RA, knee pain or gout, it's a whole lot easier, cheaper and more comfortable to restore use of your joints by the natural methods in our Arthritis Fighters than to resort to surgery or take noxious drugs for the rest of your life.

Plan Your Own Arthritis Recovery Program

Once your arthritis has been medically diagnosed, which Arthritis Fighters should you use to combat it?

For maximum benefit, I strongly advise using one or more AFs that function on the physical level (Chapter 6), one or more on the nutritional level (Chapter 7) and one or more on the psychological level (Chapter 8). This creates a whole-person approach that fights arthritis on all three levels of the body-mind at once.

I also strongly advise against flipping through this book and beginning to use an AF before you have read and understood Chapters 1 through 4. The first rule of natural healing is that before you can select and use a natural therapy intelligently, you must have at least a basic understanding of the dysfunction you are trying to heal.

By jumping straight into the middle of this book without having read the introductory chapters, you might easily use an inappropriate technique or even one that could harm your arthritis instead of helping it. Another risk is that you may fail to read cautions and caveats about who should *not* use certain therapies in this book.

Here are some guidelines to help you choose the most effective AFs for each type of arthritis. To emphasize their importance, some AFs recommended for all types of arthritis are recommended a second time for a specific type of arthritis.

FOR ALL TYPES OF ARTHRITIS

AF#1: The Eight Vital Recovery Steps That Unlock Your Inner Healing Powers

Physical Approach

AF#2: Put the Freeze on Arthritis Pain—Or Tame It with Thermotherapy

AF#3: KO Pain and Stiffness with Gentle Range-of-Motion Exercises

AF#4: Stretch Away Stiffness and Lower Back Pain

AF#5: The Amazing Benefits of Rhythmic Exercise

AF#6: Let Good Posture Help You Beat Arthritis Pain

AF#7: Let Your Muscles Ease the Agony of Arthritis

Psychological Approach

AF#15: The Funnybone Factor: Laugh Away Arthritis

AF#16: Relaxation Training: Nature's Antidote to Pain and Tension

AF#17: How to Heal Your Arthritis with Therapeutic Imagery

AF#18: Shoot Down Arthritis with Positive Beliefs

FOR RHEUMATOID ARTHRITIS—AND OTHER AUTOIMMUNE DISEASES

Nutritional Approach

AF#10: The One Diet That Does It All

AF#11: Relieve Rheumatoid Arthritis with a Natural Food from the Sea

AF#12: When Troublesome Foods May Cause "Arthritis"

AF#14: Speed Up Your Recovery with These Nutritional Heavyweights

FOR OSTEOARTHRITIS

Physical Approach

AF#5: The Amazing Benefits of Rhythmic Exercise

AF#7: Let Your Muscles Ease the Agony of Arthritis

Nutritional Approach

AF#8: Defeat Osteoarthritis by Peeling Off the Pounds

AF#9: Fewer Pounds Spell Pain-free Joints

AF#10: The One Diet That Does It All

FOR GOUT

Use the same AFs as for osteoarthritis, plus the following core Arthritis Fighters.

Nutritional Approach

AF#13: Conquer Gout without Drugs

FOR KNEE PAIN

Physical Approach

AF#5: The Amazing Benefits of Rhythmic Exercise

AF#7: Let Your Muscles Ease the Agony of Arthritis

FOR LOWER BACK PAIN

Physical Approach

AF#4: Stretch Away Stiffness and Lower Back Pain

AF#5: The Amazing Benefits of Rhythmic Exercise

AF#6: Let Good Posture Help You Beat Arthritis Pain

AF#7: Let Your Muscles Ease the Agony of Arthritis

Nutritional Approach

AF#8: Defeat Osteoarthritis by Peeling Off the Pounds

AF#9: Fewer Pounds Spell Pain-free Joints

AF#10: The One Diet That Does It All

FOR ALLERGENIC ARTHRITIS

Nutritional Approach

AF#10: The One Diet That Does It All

AF#12: When Troublesome Foods May Cause "Arthritis"

AF#14: Speed Up Your Recovery with These Nutritional Heavyweights

Add the AFs recommended for all types of arthritis to those for each specific type of arthritis, and they may add up to a dozen or more. Obviously, you can't include them all in your recovery program. So, first, select those that seem most helpful and appropriate.

Then relax. On any given level, you need perform only one or two AFs at a time. Consider the physical level AFs in Chapter 6. You can start off by using the heat and cold therapies in AF#2 and the gentle range-of-motion exercises in AF#3. As your pain diminishes and you start to limber up, you can graduate to the stretching exercises in AF#4. Then, step-by-step, you can begin to use the rhythmic exercises in AF#5 and the strength-building exercises in AF#7. As you move on into these more advanced AFs, you can drop the earlier ones.

The same thing applies to the nutritional AFs in Chapter 7. Start out with AF#8, which teaches you to assess the health of your body weight. After that, you need refer back to it only to refresh your memory. Meanwhile, progress on to the next AF in the chapter.

In the same way, as your mind and body learn to perform

the psychological AFs in Chapter 8, you will find it takes less and less time to do each one. After a few weeks of practice, many people are able to do AF#16 in just 60 seconds. Other psychological action-steps can also be carried out in just a few minutes.

What If You Have More than One Type of Arthritis?

You should also know that OA, RA and gout may all occur together. Admittedly, to have all three at once is rare. But once a joint is damaged by RA, it may develop OA as well. Some people with OA develop a low-grade fever, a symptom usually associated with RA. If you are medically diagnosed with more than one type of arthritis, you may wish to adopt AFs known to benefit both types.

The same AFs recommended for beating OA can also prevent OA. The same holds true for preventing other types of arthritis.

Once you recover from RA, you should continue to practice the same AFs that helped you recover. If, instead, you slide back into your old health-destroying habits, your arthritis is likely to return—and along with it may come other, more life-threatening diseases.

Besides helping to prevent arthritis, each of our AFs also improves your health and well-being. Make them a permanent part of your lifestyle, and you should live a long and healthful life, free of any serious disease or dysfunction.

Does the Weather Really Affect Arthritis?

Finally, in case you're wondering if the weather can affect arthritis, it probably can—but not in the way most people expect. When the weather changes from fair to stormy, people with OA claim to feel more pain in their joints, while people with RA experience weather changes throughout the body.

No proof exists that the weather directly affects arthritic joints, but some experts believe that the lack of natural light caused by stormy weather does depress our mood. As our mood drops, we experience pain more intensely. And a depression in mood is immediately mimicked by the immune system, which itself becomes depressed. This distorts its function and worsens RA.

The solution is to get outside in depressing weather and exercise if you can, all the while allowing your eyes to absorb what natural light there is. (Caution: Never look directly at the sun and wear sunglasses if your eyes are troubled by glare.)

CHAPTER SIX

The Physical Approach: Zap Arthritis Pain with Exercise

In their sixtieth year, Roy and Brenda were both afflicted with OA. Each experienced pain in one knee. Roy was afraid that exercise might damage his knee cartilage. So he retired from his job and spent his days watching TV. Month by month, his knee deteriorated until by age 63 he could barely walk.

As soon as she felt pain when climbing stairs, Brenda sought advice from a physiatrist. The physiatrist designed a daily program that included aerobic, strength-building and flexibility exercises. By her 63rd birthday, Brenda could easily walk 4 miles at a brisk pace. She could heft up a 50-pound sack of potatoes, and she could walk up and down stairs without a trace of pain.

When Brenda first saw her physiatrist, he told her that new discoveries in exercise therapy now promise a lifetime of pain-free activity for most people with arthritis. "Exercise is the best nondrug therapy in existence for relieving arthritis pain," he told Brenda. "It allows most people with arthritis to continue to function normally. In the past few months, at least fifty of my patients have replaced drugs with exercise."

But then the doctor explained that while virtually all surveys and studies have rated exercise the most successful form of arthritis treatment, the majority of arthritis patients still believe that by moving their joints they are damaging their bodies.

"The worst thing you can do for arthritis is to sit still all day watching television," the physiatrist told Brenda. "Yet most arthritis patients are willing to take any kind of drug or herb or homeopathic remedy or to wear a copper bracelet or to eat special foods. But they will not do the easy, gentle exercises recommended by the Arthritis Foundation and just about every expert on arthritis."

Don't Let Fear of Exercise Rob You of One of Nature's Best Remedies

While researching this book, I was repeatedly told by doctors and rheumatologists that a gradually increasing exercise program works better than anything else to prevent pain and disability from both OA and RA. Tens of thousands of people, for example, have discovered that walking does more to relieve the symptoms and pain of RA than any drug.

Naturally, not everyone with arthritis can walk or use strength-training machines. But almost everyone can do some kind of aerobic and strength-building exercise. If you can't walk, you can probably use your arms and hands to swim or to work out on a rowing machine. People with many forms of disability, from limbs lost in accidents to cerebral palsy or partial paralysis, manage to do isometrics or to swim, stretch or perform calisthenics.

One prominent rheumatologist helps his patients work around their limitations by focusing on activities they *can* do and not on their restrictions. It may take a while for improvement to appear, but statistics show that 95 percent of people with arthritis benefit from exercise.

Exercise: A Whole-Person Way to Heal Arthritis

Exercise creates an overall sense of well-being that benefits the entire body-mind. It replaces stress, depression, hostility, anger and anxiety with a calm but upbeat mood that lifts your spirits for the rest of the day. It sends your self-esteem soaring and restores balance to a dysfunctional immune system that may be causing RA. By enhancing strength and stamina, it raises your metabolism and keeps your weight down. It improves sleep, banishes pain and makes your joints more stable and flexible.

Most important, exercise accesses the body's healing-regeneration system. Because exercise is an active therapy, at least part of its benefits occur on the psychological level as it heals the immune system, defuses stress and releases pain-killing endorphins in the brain.

The benefits of exercise are so dependable that, even though they may not really enjoy exercising, thousands of people with arthritis force themselves to do it every day. If you don't yet have arthritis, exercise can almost totally prevent it from ever occurring. And if your arthritis symptoms are just appearing, a program of appropriate exercises may nip either OA or RA in the bud and prevent further onset.

Three Types of Exercise Benefit Arthritis

- *Aerobic*, or brisk, rhythmic exercise such as walking, bicycling or swimming keeps muscles toned and joints mobile.
- *Stretching or gentle range-of-motion exercises* such as yoga keep joints flexible and increase their mobility.
- *Strength-building exercises* increase the body's lean muscle mass, raising metabolism and burning off excess weight. These exercises also build stronger muscles which act as shock absorbers for arthritic joints, especially the knee.

The Best Time to Exercise

People with OA often feel less pain and stiffness in the morning, with discomfort increasing as the day wears on. So if you have OA, you may prefer to exercise fairly early in the day.

By contrast, people with RA may experience their worst pain in the morning. So if you have RA you may prefer to exercise in the afternoon or evening.

Whenever you exercise, the important thing is never to miss a session. Once you give in or give up, you're likely to head rapidly downhill. By skipping your exercise routine for just two or three days, your joints may become stiff and sore once more. So set aside an exercise period each day and don't allow anything to derail your plans.

Never allow lack of equipment or inability to go outdoors to stop you from exercising. You can do scores of stretching, calisthenics and isometric exercises on the living room floor and then run or step in place without anything in the way of equipment.

Nor should you put off exercising because you don't want to work out by yourself. Most health clubs, pools, gyms or senior centers offer group exercise classes for people with arthritis. With or without a companion, make exercise your top priority, as essential as sleeping or eating—not the last thing on your list!

How to Find Time to Exercise

When people tell me they can't find time to exercise, I ask how many hours a week they watch TV. Few Americans spend less than two hours a day watching the tube. That totals 14 hours, or an entire day, each week spent in a stupor hypnotized by a babbling television tube.

To beat arthritis, it helps to learn media literacy. You can break the TV habit by recognizing TV for what it really is. Virtually all commercial television exists to expose you to advertising, attracting you to watch shows that all too often depict sex and violence. Even news programs are a form of entertainment built around news items that get the highest ratings.

Cut back on TV watching, watch only shows that make you laugh, and you'll have ample time to exercise. You may also lower your risk of ever getting OA. It's an acknowledged fact that the worst thing you can do for arthritis is to sit still. OA occurs primarily in sedentary, overweight people. And that's exactly what most TV watchers become—sedentary and overweight.

Our joints don't wear out. They rust away from lack of use. As rheumatologist John H. Bland of the University of Vermont put it: "The weakest and oldest among us can become some kind of athlete. But only the strongest can survive as spectators. And only the hardiest can withstand the perils of inertia, inactivity and immobility."

Designing Your Own Program of Therapeutic Exercise

If you have arthritis, I recommend having a physical therapist or a health professional custom design an exercise program to fit your personal needs. If that isn't possible, then I suggest reading through each Arthritis Fighter in the order below and selecting what seems most appropriate.

Start with AF#2 which describes how you can remove stiffness and pain yourself with heat or cold therapy. You can apply heat or cold at any time to lessen arthritis pain or stiffness. It's also good to remember that applying heat to your joints is an excellent way to warm up before any exercise session.

AF#3 describes a series of gentle exercises that are often used to overcome stiffness and to increase mobility in arthritic joints. If you have OA or RA, you can hardly go wrong starting out with these.

As your joints become more limber, you can begin using the stretching exercises and yoga postures described in AF#4.

From there, it's just a short step to starting in on easy aerobic exercises like walking, pedaling a stationary bicycle or swimming. AF#5 introduces you to the many benefits of brisk, rhythmic exercise.

As you walk and your joints become more flexible, you can help beat arthritis by upgrading your posture. AF#6 describes how to use the famous Alexander Technique to minimize stress on muscles and joints.

Finally, AF#7 reveals how strength-training exercises can restore a full range of movement to joints afflicted with OA and, often, with RA as well.

My advice is to read each of these Arthritis Fighters in turn and use the ones you, or your doctor, believe are most appropriate for your condition. For example, avoid exercising any joint that is hot or inflamed.

Otherwise, exercise each afflicted joint for at least several minutes each day, if you can. Never push beyond the point of pain. Listen to your body and let each joint decide how far you should flex it. For instance, rowing can stress knees, while an exercise bike may be too strenuous for some people with hip or knee problems.

Start with the gentle range-of-motion exercises in AF#3. Aim to increase the mobility of your joints by using a slow, steady rhythm. Avoid any fast movement or a high number of repetitions. After exercising, rest for a period equal to the duration of your exercise session. Never exercise while taking pain-killers. And don't exercise at all until your arthritis has been medically diagnosed.

Read This Before You Start Exercising

Most health advisory services agree that, for the general public, the risk of *not* exercising far exceeds any risk of beginning a program of gradually increasing daily exercise. Most healthy men or women aged 35 or under can safely begin a daily walking program at a moderate pace. As your fitness improves, you can gradually walk a little farther and faster each day. Even so, you are cautioned never to exceed your capacity and to avoid becoming tired or fatigued. And never push yourself to the limit until you are well-conditioned.

If you are over 35, you are urged to see your doctor before starting to exercise if you have any of the following symptoms or conditions: You are a steady smoker or you consume more than two alcoholic drinks each day; you have a chronic disease or dysfunction such as heart disease, hypertension, stroke, angina, claudication or any pulmonary disease, cancer or renal disease; you are unable to walk a mile in 17.5 minutes; you are on any medication, especially beta-blockers; you experience any shortage of breath, chest pain or dizziness with or without exertion; you have diabetes or experience cuts, wounds or burns on your feet that don't heal or are slow to heal; you have lost weight during the past six months without trying; you experience fast, irregular heartbeats or very slow beats after exercise; you have osteoporosis, have fractured a hip, spine, wrist or other joint or have had a fall; or you have any orthopedic problem.

If you have one or more of these symptoms or conditions, see a doctor regardless of your age. The older and heavier you are, the more essential it is to see a physician before starting to exercise. Likewise, if you are recovering from an injury or have a disability, your physician or physical therapist should plan your exercise workouts.

These caveats apply whether or not you have arthritis. If you have arthritis in the spine, hips, knees or ankles, medical approval is essential before you start to exercise, that goes especially for brisk aerobic or strength-building exercises. Again, if you have had joint surgery or have a joint replacement, a physical therapist must design your exercise program.

A final caveat about doctors: To avoid being given biased advice by a physician who may be unfamiliar with the benefits of exercise, consult only a doctor who is obviously lean and fit and who is known to favor therapeutic exercise.

Each of the Arthritis Fighters discussed below is designed to help you fight arthritis and win.

ARTHRITIS FIGHTER #2: Put the Freeze on
Arthritis Pain — or Tame It with Thermotherapy

Applying heat or cold to an afflicted joint is one of the most effective ways to relieve the pain, stiffness or inflammation of arthritis. Although relief is temporary, it often lasts longer than that provided by pain-killing drugs. And both heat and cold therapy are safe, cheap and free of side effects.

Which is best? Heat or cold?

That depends. Heat, or thermotherapy, soothes and relieves pain and stiffness due to either OA or RA. But it should never be used when there is inflammation, heat, redness or swelling—all symptoms usually associated with RA.

Applying heat to an afflicted joint relaxes muscles and arteries so that stiffness melts away and blood flow increases. Since the cells, platelets, enzymes and hormones that form the body's healing-regeneration system are all carried by the bloodstream, increased blood supply is a natural way to speed the healing process. Thus, heat swiftly relaxes a stiffened joint and restores flexibility and mobility.

Heat is particularly helpful upon first awakening when people with arthritis often experience stiffness and pain. Many people also find that soaking in a warm bath for 15 to 20 minutes is a great way to limber up before starting to exercise.

Never apply heat to any one area for more than 20 to 25 minutes nor on any area you've just rubbed with a heat-producing cream such as Ben Gay. Never apply heat to a joint that is red, swollen or inflamed. Always apply a heating pad *over* a joint, never *under* it. If you fall asleep lying on a heating pad, you could be badly burned. The heat source you use should be between 98.6° and 105° F. If you have hypertension, you should not use a whirlpool, jacuzzi or sauna without medical approval.

Provided you have no sign of inflammation or swelling, most physical therapists I've talked with suggest trying heat first. If that doesn't work, they suggest trying cold.

When Cold May Work Better than Heat

Applying cold, or cryotherapy, to an afflicted area reduces blood flow and is usually recommended for a hot inflamed joint, for gout or bursitis or for any muscle that is aching or overused. Cold eases pain by reducing joint temperature, it penetrates more deeply than heat, and it is believed to stimulate endorphin production. Several researchers have confirmed that cold inhibits transmission of nerve impulses to the brain's pain center and that cold is an effective analgesic for RA pain.

Cold has proven particularly successful at relieving the pain of RA in the knees. For example, when Dr. Peter Utsinger of Germantown Hospital in Philadelphia had 24 people with painful knees place an icepack above and below the knees for 20 minutes three times each day, virtually every person showed significant improvement in range of motion, sleep, pain and other functions after a month of therapy. In another study, Dr. Utsinger had 240 people with arthritis and knee pain apply icebags to their afflicted joints once each day. At the end of a month, 85 percent reported decreased pain and reduced inflammation. Overall, Dr. Utsinger found that cold often worked well when heat did not and that cold proved an acceptable substitute for oral analgesics.

Every drugstore carries a selection of icebags as well as refreezable gel-filled pads. Gel pads can be cooled in a freezer and moulded around the painful joint. To use cryotherapy on a knee, for example, use two gel pads, one above and one below the painful area, and secure both pads with an elastic bandage.

If nothing else is available, you can place a bag of frozen peas on a painful joint to numb it. The peas will mould themselves around the joint. Or you can use a strong plastic bag filled with ice cubes or crushed ice and covered with a thin towel.

A word of caution before you begin: Take care not to apply cold to any one area for more than 15 minutes at a time and not more frequently than once every 4.5 hours. Always place a cloth between the cold source and the skin to prevent frostbite.

If neither heat nor cold helps ease your pain and stiffness, you could have a fracture or an injured ligament or tendon. In that case, I recommend seeing a doctor.

Amazing Benefits from Moist Heat

Moist heat is most effective for relieving the pain of an acute RA flare-up (dry heat penetrates more deeply and is best for applying deep heat to a joint). In either case, heat is a powerful pain reliever and results are often dramatic.

Nowadays, drugstores carry a variety of electrically powered moist or dry heating pads. Or moist heat can be applied with a simple, homemade hot compress. Crumple a loaf of cheap, white bread inside a thick, folded towel and soak it in hot water at roughly 116°F. Wring out the towel and wrap it immediately over the afflicted joint. Cover the towel with waxed paper and wrap a dry towel around that. Known as a bread compress, it will hold heat longer than a towel alone. Any type of homemade hot compress must be resoaked in hot water and reapplied every few minutes.

You can easily apply moist heat to feet, ankles, hands or wrists by immersing them in a bucket of warm water or by placing them in a small tub or footbath. For best results, the water should be 6 inches above the ankles or wrists. Water temperature should be close to 105°F and you should immerse the hands or feet for 5 full minutes at a time.

A steamroom is an excellent way to apply soothing heat to the whole body. Alternately, relaxing for 15 to 20 minutes in a tub of warm to moderately hot water provides soothing relaxation to every joint in the body. A number of people tell me that they mix 2 cups of Epsom salts in the water, while others add bath oil or bubbles. A whirlpool or jacuzzi bath also provides a water massage and can benefit almost every case of arthritis.

If you only have a shower, spray moderately hot water on the painful area for 6 minutes, then spray your neck, shoulders, back and scalp for an additional 5 minutes. After that, alternate between the two at 1-minute intervals for another 9 minutes. Try to stay in the shower a total of 20 minutes.

Any type of bath will supply a whole-body moist heat treatment that relaxes every muscle simultaneously. Many people take a hot bath as soon as they wake up and do some of their range-of-motion exercises while in the water.

Dry Heat Goes Deepest

Dry heat is often the most effective way to apply deep heat to relieve the pain in a joint afflicted with OA. Almost any electric heating pad or heat lamp will supply dry heat. Make sure that the lamp heats by infrared rays and not ultraviolet. Place the lamp 2 feet from the body and focus the rays on the painful area for 20 to 25 minutes.

An electric blanket also supplies dry heat. Several people report using a timer to turn on their electric blanket 1 hour before waking. The warmth relieves early morning stiffness without creating too much heat during the night.

For a makeshift dry heating pad, fill an old sock with any type of uncooked rice and close the top of the sock securely with a cord. Heat the sock in a microwave for 3 minutes. Test the heat before you apply the pad to a joint, and then place it over the joint. It will immediately adapt to the shape of the joint and will hold heat for up to 1 hour. Since microwave settings vary, you may have to experiment a few times to get the right temperature. Gel pads can also be warmed in a microwave.

To apply dry heat to the whole body, a sauna is best.

Blessed Relief from Paraffin Wax

Coating the toes or fingers with hot paraffin wax has long been a popular way of applying dry heat uniformly to arthritic joints in the hands or feet. The entire hand or foot is dipped several times into molten wax in a paraffin bath. It sets and hardens immediately. The hand or foot is then covered with a plastic bag and heated towels. The wax supplies 15 to 20 minutes of deep, soothing heat and relaxation. Because the wax contains mineral oil, it peels off easily when cool.

While it is true that many people prepare and use their own hot wax baths, almost all have been trained to do so by a physical therapist. Without proper instruction, you could easily burn yourself or upset the wax pot and start a fire. Thus, I urge you to have a physical therapist demonstrate the correct way to prepare and use the wax before you attempt it on your own.

Physical therapists and other health professionals can also provide deep-heat treatment using ultrasound. The ultrasound waves penetrate deep into a joint and heat up small areas. Records show that ultrasound treatment helps 80 percent of arthritis patients. Although it's possible to buy ultrasound equipment, the consensus of medical opinion is that it's safer to have a physical therapist provide the treatment.

Sleeping Warm Eliminates Early Morning Stiffness

Another aspect of thermotherapy was confirmed some years ago in tests at St. Margaret's Hospital in Pittsburgh when researchers found that sleeping warm and snug is a proven way to prevent the morning pain, stiffness and swelling associated with RA.

Wearing unlined stretch medical gloves while sleeping, it was found, effectively relieves morning stiffness in the hands. The gloves, available in drug, department or medical stores, work by both warming the hands and exerting pressure on hands and wrists.

Another good way to sleep warm is to use a sleeping bag. Researchers have found a bag far superior to an electric blanket. In recent surveys, hundreds of people with RA who sleep in warm sleeping bags reported they had almost completely eliminated morning stiffness. The next best thing to a sleeping bag is wearing thermal underwear and white cotton or wool socks in bed. Be sure to buy thermal underwear two sizes too large since it shrinks.

You can also keep joints warm during sleep by wrapping them in thermoelastic products made of Spandex or similar material. Tube-shaped they can be slipped over a hand or foot to keep knees and elbows warm.

Tips on Sleeping Well

Anyone with RA needs more sleep and rest during flare-ups and less rest and more activity during remissions. Try to sleep at least 8 to 9 hours each night during flare-ups. You may also sleep better during flare-ups if you take an afternoon nap of 20 minutes to 2 hours.

During remissions, you will sleep better if you avoid naps and consolidate sleep into a single nighttime unit. At all costs, avoid extended bed rest. Excessive periods of inactivity can stiffen joints and weaken muscles.

During RA flare-ups, the most comfortable way to sleep is lying flat on your back with all limbs and joints straight but relaxed. Try to keep knees, hips, elbows, wrists, fingers and toes straight. Have your arms at your sides with palms up, and try to avoid bending or curling any joint. Do not place pillows under your knees as that may leave you with stiff, bent joints. But you can use folded towels under ankles, wrists and arms to help keep them straight.

If you must change position, lie on your side with your knees drawn up. Keep your neck and head in line with your spine by using only one average-sized pillow.

ARTHRITIS FIGHTER #3: KO Pain and Stiffness with Gentle Range-of-Motion Exercises

---

Arthritis is loss of movement in a joint due to pain, stiffness and muscle atrophy. You can take all the prescription drugs, herbs or homeopathic remedies ever devised, but you won't recover from arthritis until you can move that joint once more through its maximum possible range of motion without stiffness or pain.

According to top rheumatologists, a series of stretching movements known as "gentle range-of-motion exercises" work better than anything else to prevent pain and stiffness and to restore flexibility and movement to a joint afflicted with arthritis. These exercises were specifically designed to put each body joint through its complete range of motion. Experience has shown that, in the process, the exercises relieve pain better than most drugs and with no side effects.

In an arthritic joint, inflammation, swelling and cartilage damage create pain and stiffness that limit a joint's range of motion. When moving a joint is painful, we tend not to move it beyond the point of pain. Once we stop exercising a joint, synovial fluid is no longer excreted and the cartilage is deprived of nutrients. The muscles that work that joint weaken and atrophy, and flabby muscles increase the risk of injury to any joint, especially the knees. When this happens, a joint becomes increasingly stiff and painful, and its range of movement becomes extremely limited.

By improving the circulation of blood, lymph and synovial fluid to an arthritic joint, stretching restores freedom of movement and prevents further shortening of muscles. The simple range-of-motion exercises described below are the first step toward helping your joints limber up and move without pain. With a little perseverance, you can then continue on to more advanced yoga stretching and to aerobic and strength-building exercises that enable most people with arthritis to begin functioning normally once more.

When and for How Long Should You Exercise?

Ideally, you should strive for a total of 15 minutes of range-of-motion exercise each day. If you like, you can begin while still warm in bed in the morning, perhaps in a sleeping bag or under an electric blanket. It's easy to move your fingers, wrists, elbows, ankles and knees for a few minutes while under the covers. People who do usually find it easier to get up. Others take a warm bath as soon as they get up and do as many exercises as possible while immersed in the water.

While most people prefer to exercise during a single 15-minute period as early in the day as possible, others report good results by exercising 3 times a day for 5 minutes. Later in the day, if your wrists and fingers are stiff, try immersing them in warm water for 2 to 3 minutes before exercising.

For best results, exercise each joint in the body for a few minutes each day. Move slowly and gently and never beyond the point of pain. Never exercise a joint that is inflamed, red, hot or swollen. Don't worry if you can't move your joint far enough to complete the movement described in the exercise. Begin by doing what you can and keep exercising regularly. Gradually, your joint should become more flexible until you can move it through its maximum possible range of motion.

At least a hundred different therapeutic exercises have been developed to help unfreeze arthritic joints. (For information about others, contact the Arthritis Foundation listed in the appendix. It also has videos demonstrating each exercise.) For the average person with arthritis, the stretches described below are probably most beneficial.

Start off with a few, then add one new exercise each day to your repertoire. Even if your joints are not all stiff, exercising nonarthritic joints can prevent arthritis from developing there.

TO UNFREEZE A STIFF NECK

Sit in an upright chair with both feet flat on the floor and hands on thighs.

Step 1. Keep your head level like a Thai dancer. Pull your chin back as far as possible to make a double chin. Then slide your head all the way forward and stick your chin out. Repeat 10 times.

Step 2. Tilt your head up and back as far as you can. Then gently drop your chin to your chest and lower your head as much as you can.

Step 3. Slowly tilt and stretch your head down to the right, trying to touch your right shoulder with your right ear. Then

115

repeat to the left. Try not to bend your head forward. Repeat 5 times on each side.

Step 4. Keeping your head and neck erect, rotate your head slowly to the right as far as you can and look back over your right shoulder. Then repeat to the left. Do the exercise twice on each side.

Step 5. Relax your neck and slowly do a neck roll. Starting with your chin down on your chest, roll your head all the way to the right, then all the way back, then all the way to the left and finally back down on your chest. Do 3 complete rolls in each direction.

You can use these movements to stretch your neck while at work, while typing or while watching TV.

TO UNFREEZE STIFF FINGERS AND WRISTS

Exercise 1. Exercise your thumb joints by repeatedly touching the tip of your thumb to the base of the little finger on the same hand. Next, clench both fists and hold tightly squeezed for 5 seconds. Then open both hands and stretch fingers and thumbs as wide as possible for 5 seconds.

With fingers straight, bend your wrists back as far as you can. Hold for 5 seconds and release. Then open both hands as wide as you can. Finally, bend both wrists sideways as far as you can in each direction. Repeat the entire exercise 5 times.

Exercise 2. If your wrists are stiff, place your palms and fingers together in front of you as if praying. Press the left hand backwards with the right hand so that the left wrist bends back. Then repeat in the other direction. Push each wrist back just past the point of discomfort and hold for 5 seconds. Repeat 5 times with each wrist.

116

Exercise 3. To increase strength and flexibility in your fingers, stretch out your arm and hold the corner of a double page of newspaper. Crumple up the page into a small ball using only one hand. Repeat 5 times with each hand. Typing, especially on a computer, or playing the piano also helps restore flexibility to stiff fingers and wrists.

If your fingers are chronically stiff from OA, consider learning the American Manual Alphabet. This hand-performed sign language, used by people unable to hear or speak, requires dexterous use of fingers and wrists. Several rheumatologists have recommended it for restoring range of motion to every joint in the fingers and hands. However, it is not recommended for those with RA.

TO UNFREEZE STIFF SHOULDERS

Exercise 1. Stand or sit in an upright position. Raise one shoulder as high as you can and drop it as low as you can. Repeat with the other shoulder. Then raise and lower both shoulders together as if you were shrugging. Next, roll both shoulders in one direction 5 times and roll them in the opposite direction 5 times. If you can move only one shoulder at a time, do the same exercises using one shoulder.

Exercise 2. Stand or sit in an upright position. Extend both arms straight out in front of you and keep both arms and wrists straight. Trace small circles in the air with your hands, first in one direction, then in the other. Gradually make the circles as large as you can. Finally, keep your arms still while you rotate your hands and wrists as far as they will go in one direction and then as far as possible in the other direction.

Next, stretch both arms out sideways and repeat the same movements. Lastly, raise your arms overhead and repeat the same movements.

Exercise 3. With your elbows at your waist, move them back as far as you can so that your shoulder blades are pinched together. Repeat 3 times.

Exercise 4. Stand upright with your legs straight and about 12 inches apart. Hold on to a chair with one hand for support. Bend forward from the waist. Let your free arm hang down so that your hand dangles loosely near the floor. Start to trace small circles with your hand, first in one direction, then the other. As your shoulder warms up, make the circles larger. Change over and repeat with the other hand. Then return to the upright position.

Exercise 5. Stand or sit in an upright position. Extend your arms straight out sideways at shoulder height. Keeping your arms straight, move them forward until your palms touch. Still keeping your arms fully extended at shoulder height, move them back behind you as far as you can. Return your arms so they are extended straight out at your sides. Then lower them until they are hanging at your sides. Lastly, raise both arms overhead as high as you can. If possible, touch your hands together over your head. Then release. Repeat the entire exercise 3 times.

TO UNFREEZE STIFF ELBOWS

Exercise 1. Stand or sit in an upright position. Clasp your hands together in front of you. Bend your elbows and bring your clasped hands up to your left shoulder. Continue to move your hands up and over your shoulder as far as you can.

Next, straighten your elbows and bring your clasped hands to your right knee. Then bring your clasped hands to your right shoulder and back down to your left knee. If you can't do it all, do what you can. Repeat the entire exercise 5 times.

Exercise 2. Place your right hand on your right shoulder, and your left hand on your left shoulder, with elbows extended out to the sides. Next, extend both arms out to your sides until the elbows are straight. Return both hands to your shoulders. Repeat 10 times.

TO UNFREEZE A STIFF WAIST

Exercise 1. Stand upright with your hands on your hips. Keep your feet, legs and hips as still as possible. Try to avoid rotating your hips. Then turn your head, trunk, and arms slowly all the way to the right and keep twisting as far as you can go to your right. Hold 10 seconds, then return to center. Repeat the same exercise to the left. Do 3 repetitions in each direction.

Exercise 2. Lie on your back on the floor on a rug or carpet. Keep your feet flat on the floor, with your knees bent. Keeping your shoulders and back on the floor, slowly twist your hips to the left as far as you can until your knees touch the floor. Hold 5 seconds and return to the starting position. Then twist the same way to the right and return. Repeat twice in each direction.

TO UNFREEZE STIFF KNEES AND HIPS

Lie on your back on a rug on the floor with your legs straight. Raise one knee, bending it at the knee and hip, and bring it toward your chest until both knee and hip are bent as far as possible. Next, straighten your knee and slowly lower your leg back to the floor. Repeat with the other leg.

119

Do as many repetitions as you can with each leg up to a maximum of 10.

TO UNFREEZE STIFF ANKLES AND FEET

Exercise 1. Lie on your back on a rug on the floor with your legs straight and your feet about 15 inches apart. Rotate your ankles sideways, first all the way outwards, then all the way inwards. Next, using your ankles, point both feet down and away from you as far as you can. Finally, raise your toes up and toward you as far as you can. Repeat each movement 10 times.

Exercise 2. One of the best ways to exercise your feet is to sit in a chair and roll an empty bottle back and forth on the floor with one foot. Then, to free up the toes, place some large ball bearings or marbles on the floor and try to pick them up, one by one, with your toes.

Flexing Your Joints in a Warm Swimming Pool

Gentle range-of-motion exercises have proven so helpful in freeing up stiff joints that almost every exercise facility with a warm water swimming pool offers regular exercise classes for people with arthritis. For best results, the pool temperature should be between 88 and 90°F. A cooler temperature may fail to warm stiff joints, while a warmer temperature may be dangerous for people with cardiovascular problems.

If you have access to such a pool, but classes are not available, you can easily work out your own exercise routine. Begin by flexing your fingers and toes, then your ankles, wrists, knees and hips. Slowly rotate and stretch any joints afflicted with arthritis. Then stretch and rotate every other joint as far as you can, including your neck. To end your session, try walking backward waist deep in the pool.

ARTHRITIS FIGHTER #4: Stretch Away Stiffness and Lower Back Pain

Once you can do the more advanced range-of-motion exercises in AF#3, it's just a short step into yoga, the *ultimate* range-of-motion therapy.

Although most of us may recognize yoga as a type of stretching exercise developed 2,000 years ago in India, yoga is actually a whole-person way of achieving total health. Yoga includes not only stretches and postures that restore flexibility and a full range of motion to stiff joints but also a health-building diet and system of stress management based on meditation.

One woman I knew who developed RA at age 44 adopted the entire yoga philosophy and lifestyle. While she stretched away stiffness from her joints, she also became a strict vegetarian and eliminated stress from her life by meditating for 20 minutes each day.

It took about 4 months for this combination of therapies to beat her RA. From then on, she experienced a total remission. That was more than 5 years ago, and her RA symptoms have never returned. The reason is, of course, that she has continued to faithfully practice yoga on a whole-person level without missing a single day. Doing so has mobilized and maintained her body's healing-regeneration system in exactly the way I described in Chapter 2.

Revitalize Your Joints with Yoga

Yoga can be powerful medicine for any type of arthritis (I'm only going to cover the physical aspects of yoga here). One survey found that 90 percent of people with OA or RA who practiced yoga stretches regularly received significant

121

benefits. For those who suffered from lower back pain—itself a type of arthritis—more than 90 percent recovered completely and had no further problems with their backs.

Actually, all modern range-of-motion exercises are based on yoga. Some have been simplified, and the original Sanskrit names have been made easier to pronounce. But essentially they are all based on centuries-old yoga stretching postures called *"asanas."* At least 30 of the best-known asanas are used today for increasing flexibility and relieving pain in arthritic joints.

There are two ways to stretch. *Ballistic* stretching is achieved by fast, repetitive bouncing. Understandably, this is not the best treatment for arthritic joints.

Static stretching, by contrast, means slowly stretching a joint through its full existing range of motion until you meet pain or resistance. At this point, you back off very slightly and hold the stretch for up to 2 minutes before letting go. Static stretching is far more effective for arthritis and much less likely to cause injury.

Hatha yoga is a method of static stretching in which asanas are performed slowly and held from 10 to 30 seconds, or up to 2 minutes, while you continue to breathe at a relaxed pace. Since diet and stress management are covered in other Arthritis Fighter techniques later in the book, I shall focus on performing and practicing hatha yoga asanas here.

How Yoga Helps Heal and Rehabilitate Arthritic Joints

Provided you adopt diet and meditation along with the asanas, yoga may help you achieve a total remission from RA. The mere physical act of performing the asanas can also release the healing powers of the mind. While you breathe, stretch and balance as you perform asanas to limber up the body, you may also find you are calming the mind and letting go of stress—a classic example of the intimate link between body and mind.

Arthritis isn't the only way to make a joint stiff. Sedentary living works just as well. In fact, stiffness in a joint can be due as much to lack of use as to arthritis. From the moment we stop using a joint, the muscles shorten, cartilage dries out and the joint becomes stiff and rapidly loses its full range of motion.

The result is chronic stiffness, a degenerative condition that impairs agility and coordination and eventually leads to the familiar limp and stiff gait that we associate with arthritis. In sedentary people, spinal rigidity and joint stiffness often appear by age 30, and this form of premature aging worsens each year.

Recent studies have shown that whether restricted mobility is due to arthritis, sedentary living or both, you can win back much of your youthful flexibility. By exercising regularly with hatha yoga, you can break the collagen links that stiffen joints and restore elasticity to your limbs and spine.

Stop Lower Back Pain Now with Yoga

Every day, lower back pain keeps more than 6 million Americans in bed or incapacitated. After age 45, this form of arthritis becomes a recurring problem for 1 in every 3 Americans. In most cases, the problem becomes progressively worse and occurs more frequently with age. No wonder, when you consider the spine is the most complex system of joints in the body. Though we tend to blame a ruptured spinal disc for chronic back pain, most cases are due to a combination of weak back and abdominal muscles, unresolved emotional stress and being overweight.

As the Texas Back Institute advises, "The best weapon to fight off back pain is not a pill, bed rest, heating pad or hocus pocus. It's simply a stronger and more flexible back." Most people with chronic back pain have back and hamstring muscles that are too tight for toe touching and abdominal muscles that are too weak to do sit-ups.

However, most cases of lower back pain are classic examples of physical dysfunction that is psychological in origin. To start with, most back pain is not caused by damage to the spinal vertebrae or cartilage. It is directly triggered by unresolved emotional stress coupled with weak, flabby muscles in the abdomen and back.

For example, when you're suddenly struck by an excruciating pain in your lower back as you raise a window at bedtime, your pain may have more to do with an argument you had with your boss 10 hours earlier than with the muscular effort of raising the window.

What actually happens is that a stressful event, such as a confrontation with the boss in midafternoon, triggers the fight-or-flight response and tenses all the muscles for emergency action. When a person can neither fight nor flee, the tension proves too much for poorly conditioned, unused muscles. They go into spasm, and the slightest exertion may cause a tiny tear in overtaut back muscles. This microtear is all it takes to set off a piercing jolt of pain in the lower back. For the next few days, every movement of the spine feels like a dozen red-hot knives stabbing deep into your lower back.

Once any medical or orthopedic problem has been ruled out by a doctor, most cases of lower back pain respond well to yoga postures designed to stretch back muscles. Several years ago, a survey of back pain patients by New York market researcher Arthur C. Klein concluded that yoga produced the best, most successful long-term relief for lower back pain.

For recovery to be complete, however, two other action-steps must be fulfilled. First, weak abdomen and back muscles must be strengthened by performing some of the strength-training exercises described in AF#7. Second, see AF#8 for a weight-loss program that really works. Being overweight and having a protruding abdomen is another prominent cause of lower back pain. Every 10 pounds of surplus fat on the abdomen throws a strain of 50 extra pounds on the back muscles each time they are moved.

Yoga alone can't prevent lower back pain from recurring until these two major health problems have also been rectified. Then, by elongating the spine and developing flexibility, the recommended yoga asanas described below should relieve much of the stiffness in the abdomen, hip, hamstring and back extensor muscles that predispose a person to lower back pain.

How to Begin Using Yoga

By far the best and safest way is to enroll in a beginning hatha yoga class conducted by an experienced instructor who will start you off at a gentle level. Tell the instructor that you have arthritis in certain joints. Since yoga is entirely noncompetitive, simply do what you can without pushing yourself to the point of pain or discomfort. An experienced instructor will see that you perform each asana correctly so that you don't overstretch a joint and temporarily set back recovery of its range of motion.

For this reason, no one with arthritis should attempt to practice even the most elementary posture without a physician's approval. This caveat is especially important if a joint is swollen or inflamed by RA. It also applies whether you enroll in a class, teach yourself yoga or try some of the stretches described below.

Most classes are nominally priced, and once you learn the postures, you can continue doing them at home. However, many people prefer the support of a group and the discipline and regularity of a class. It's true that most yoga teachers and students are women, but most men find yoga at least as challenging as working out with weights.

All you need is a pair of tights, shorts or leotards and a blanket or mat. I recommend purchasing a "sticky" mat, which is a special nonslip rubber mat designed to hold your hands and feet in place while practicing yoga.

Yoga Is Free for the Doing

If you can't attend a yoga class, consider teaching yourself from a book or videotape. Among the most helpful books is *The Art of Living* by Rene Taylor (Keats Publishing) plus *Integral Yoga Hatha* by Swami Satchidananda and *The Complete Illustrated Book of Yoga* by Swami Vishnudevananda. The last two, both yoga classics, can be found in most libraries. Once you have learned the basic asanas, I recommend *Yoga: The Iyengar Way* by Mira Silva and Shyam Mehta (Knopf, 1990). B. K. S. Iyengar is an Indian yoga teacher who modified the asanas of traditional hatha yoga into his own personalized system. Most Iyengar yoga postures are extremely helpful in limbering up stiff joints, and Iyengar yoga is currently the most popular form of hatha yoga taught in America.

Among videotapes for beginners, I like *Forever Flexible* with Lilias Folan, *Yoga Journal*'s *Yoga Practice for Beginners* with Patricia Walden and *Easy Yoga for Seniors* with

Pat Laster. *Yoga Journal* (see Appendix) is an excellent source of current yoga books and tapes and of places to purchase sticky mats. The magazine's Book and Tape Service stocks and sells many yoga books and tapes, including *Yoga Journal*'s three practice tapes featuring Patricia Walden.

Getting Started

However you begin, ease into yoga gradually and don't attempt any advanced postures until you have mastered the easier ones first. Always warm up your joints before performing hatha yoga by walking briskly and swinging the arms for 6 to 8 minutes.

Breathe normally while stretching and don't hold the breath. Keep the back straight at all times unless you're actually flexing the spine. Perform each posture in a slow, relaxed way. Stretch gradually through the full range of motion until you meet resistance and feel mild discomfort. At that point, back off slightly and hold the stretch for at least 10 seconds. As you become more flexible, gradually increase the time up to 1 or 2 minutes. Stop immediately if pain occurs and avoid that stretch until you're fully recovered. Then begin again at a gentle level. Above all, continue to practice or attend class regularly 2 to 3 times a week.

Be aware that benefits last only for as long as you continue to practice yoga regularly. For example, 15 minutes a day for 4 days a week is better than 1 hour once a week. And while you can maintain flexibility with aerobic exercise, hatha yoga is still the best way to restore and preserve a joint's full range of motion.

Hatha yoga will improve stiffness, whether it's due to arthritis, lower back pain, sedentary living or any other reason. But to relieve stiffness due to arthritis or lower back pain, the following basic asanas are considered among the most beneficial.

Salute to the Sun	Cat and Dog Stretch*
The Cobra*	Forward Bending Pose*
The Locust*	Knee-to-Chest Curl*
Upper Back Stretch*	Spinal Twist*
Plow	Fish Pose
Pelvic Pose*	Triangle Pose

Unfortunately, lack of space prevents describing how to do every one of these helpful postures. But here, to get you started, are brief instructions for performing eight of the hatha yoga asanas (those noted with a *) listed above. (Before you try them, read the caveats under "How to Begin Using Yoga" and, near the beginning of the chapter, "Read This Before You Start Exercising.")

THE COBRA

By stretching the spine backwards, this classic yoga posture opens up space between the vertebrae, increases circulation to bones and tissue, counteracts the forward slouch that results from sitting all day and gives a good stretch to the quadricep muscles.

Step 1. Lie face down on a rug on the floor. Your legs should be straight and together, toenails facing down. Place your hands beneath your shoulders, palms down. Keep your buttock muscles tight to protect your back.
Step 2. As you inhale, use your back muscles to raise your

head, neck and shoulders as high as possible. Then use your arms to continue raising your chest off the floor, arching your spine back. Next, raise your head as high as you can, tilting it back and looking up. Keep your abdomen and pelvis flat on the floor.

Hold for 5 to 10 seconds as you breathe deeply. Return to the floor slowly as you exhale. As your spine becomes more flexible, you'll be able to go higher and hold the asana for a longer period.

THE LOCUST

This posture prevents lower back pain by giving a good stretch to the lumbar extensor muscles in the lower back. It also strengthens the lower back muscles.

Step 1. Lie face down on a rug on the floor. Clench your fists loosely, and with knuckles down, place them under your hips.

Step 2. Keeping your right leg straight, slowly raise it as high in the air as you can while you inhale. Hold it for 6 seconds, breathing normally, and lower it back to the floor as you exhale. Repeat with the left leg. Continue to alternate up to 10 times with each leg. As your range of motion increases, raise each leg higher and hold for as long as you can. For greater comfort, try placing a pillow under your pelvis.

Step 3. As you become stronger, raise both legs at once. Keep them straight and together and raise them as high as you can. Hold for 6 seconds, then slowly lower as you exhale. Gradually raise the legs higher and hold the asana for up to 2 minutes.

129

UPPER BACK STRETCH

By stretching the upper back muscles, this asana prevents a recurrence of lower back pain.

Step 1. Lie on your back on a rug on the floor. Place your arms at your sides with palms down. Bend your knees, keeping your feet flat on the floor.
Step 2. Cross your right leg over your left leg.
Step 3. Twist your torso all the way around to the right while turning your shoulders as far to the right as you can and turning your head to look over your right shoulder.
Hold the position for 10 seconds or longer. Repeat on the other side. Then do the stretch up to 4 more times in each direction.

PELVIC POSE

This is a splendid asana for restoring range of motion to hips, knees and ankles.

Step 1. Kneel on a rug on the floor with your feet extended so that your toenails are facing down. (Your entire lower leg, from knee to toes, should be resting on the floor.) Keep the knees together.
Step 2. Slowly sit back on your legs until your heels and buttocks touch.
Step 3. Bend your trunk and shoulders forward until your forehead touches the floor. Stretch your arms over your head with your palms touching the floor.
Hold this position for up to 2 minutes while breathing normally throughout. Then return to a sitting position.

CAT AND DOG STRETCH

This is a splendid asana for removing spinal stiffness and for stretching the back and abdominal muscles.

Step 1. Get on your hands and knees on a rug on the floor. Your back should be parallel to the floor.

Step 2. Inhale deeply. As you exhale, arch your back as high as possible like an angry cat. Simultaneously, drop your head and neck as low as you can while you tuck in your chin and suck in your abdomen toward your spine.

Hold this pose for the 5-to-8-second duration of your exhalation.

Step 3. As you inhale, reverse the stance and make like a dog looking up at the sky. Relax your abdomen and fill it with air as you inhale. Looking up raise your neck, head and chin up as high as you can and flex your spine to create a caved-in hollow in the small of your back. Hold this posture throughout the 5-to-8 seconds of your exhalation.

Step 4. Without bouncing or losing momentum, repeat the entire exercise up to 10 times in rhythm with your breathing.

FORWARD BENDING POSE (OR BACK OR HAMSTRING STRETCH)

By touching the toes with legs straight, this asana provides a good stretch to hips, spine, shoulders and hamstring muscles.

Step 1. Sit on a rug on the floor with your legs together and fully extended. Breathe normally throughout.

Step 2. As you inhale, stretch your arms overhead and lengthen your spine.

Step 3. As you exhale, bend forward and reach your hands out toward your toes. Try to grasp your left toe with your left hand and your right toe with your right hand. If you cannot reach your toes, grasp your ankles or lower legs. Keep your knees straight, your legs flat on the floor and your ankles relaxed. Bend your elbows if you can, and use your arms to pull yourself forward. Hold the pose 10 seconds or longer. Relax and repeat twice more. Then with your arms still raised overhead, return to a sitting position and lower your arms to the floor.

KNEE-TO-CHEST CURL

While relieving and preventing lower back pain, this asana improves range of motion in knees, hips, neck, elbows and shoulders.

Step 1. Lie on your back on a rug on the floor with your knees raised and your feet on the floor about 12 inches apart.

Step 2. Raise both knees together, clasp your hands around them and pull your knees into your chest. Hold this position as you inhale. Then, as you exhale, crunch your head, neck and shoulders up off the floor while keeping your lower back flat on the rug. Hold for several seconds and release. Repeat this step 4 more times.

SPINAL TWIST

This simple twist helps relieve and prevent lower back pain while increasing range of motion in the spine and neck.

Step 1. Sit sideways on a straight-backed chair with your left hip against the back of the chair. Keep your back straight, knees and legs together and feet flat on the floor.

Step 2. Turn your shoulders left toward the back of the chair. Place your hands on top of the chair back, one hand at each end. Pull with the right hand, drawing your right shoulder around toward the chair back. Push with your left hand to turn your left shoulder around and away from the back of the chair. Turn your head to the left as far as you can and look over your left shoulder. Keep trying to turn your hips, shoulders, neck and head around to the left as far as you can. Hold for up to 30 seconds or longer. Then relax and repeat on the other side.

Step 3. Finish the pose by sitting on the front of the chair. Spread your knees apart and drop your head down between your knees while relaxing your spine, neck and head for 10 seconds or longer. Then slowly raise back up to a sitting position.

The best way to keep arthritis at bay is to move every joint in the body through its full range of motion at least once each day.

ARTHRITIS FIGHTER #5: The Amazing Benefits of Rhythmic Exercise

---

Fifty-five-year-old Phyllis had RA so badly in her knees that her doctor was considering total knee replacement surgery. But Phyllis was terrified of hospitals and operations. When she read that walking was one of the best ways to relieve the pain and stiffness of arthritis, she decided to give it a try. With her doctor's approval, Phyllis bought a pair of well-cushioned walking shoes and embarked on a program of gradually increasing daily walks. She also began a series of exercises to restore strength to the muscles in her knees and thighs.

Her knees were so stiff that to walk at all was painful at first. But as Phyllis persevered, the pain in her knees gradually diminished. By her sixteenth week, she was walking 3 miles a day, and except during an occasional flare-up, her arthritis pain had almost disappeared.

"Whenever I have a flare-up I know that only walking can defuse the pain," she told me during an interview. "So I find myself walking when my pain is at its worst. But walking never fails. Within an hour the pain is gone. Walking sure beats any pain medication and it leaves no side effects."

Phyllis's case isn't an isolated instance.

Studies at the Washington University Arthritis Center in St. Louis confirmed that a brisk daily walk—or any equivalent rhythmic exercise—reduced all forms of arthritis pain. In one study of 102 patients with OA of the knee (reported in *Annals of Internal Medicine,* April 1, 1992), researchers found that after taking part in a regular walking exercise program for two months, most participants reported a considerable reduction in pain and they used far fewer pain medications than a control group that did not exercise.

Tame Arthritis with Aerobic Exercise

Granted, not everyone with arthritis can walk. Yet similar results occur with *any* type of brisk, rhythmic exercise. Whether you pedal a stationary bicycle, swim or use a rowing machine, 35 minutes of brisk movement turns on the natural feel-good mechanism in our brain. Millions of tiny morphine-like molecules called "endorphins" are released. Each endorphin binds on to a pain receptor in the brain and, either fully or partially, blocks out most of the sensation of arthritis pain.

Rhythmic exercise like walking, swimming or bicycling is also known as aerobic exercise, meaning that it employs the body's large muscle groups in a brisk, continuous and unbroken rhythm sufficiently vigorous to raise the heartbeat, breathing rate and oxygen uptake. By comparison, stop-and-go exercises like walking a golf course provide few, if any, aerobic benefits.

True aerobic exercise benefits every cell, muscle and joint in the body. It improves posture, balance and muscle tone, relieves tension and stress, restores cardiovascular fitness, builds stamina and endurance and strengthens the immune system, reducing risk of cancer or infection.

Aerobic exercise is especially beneficial for people with arthritis. By increasing joint mobility it lessens stiffness and combats pain. It brings more blood to muscles in joints, and it feeds more nutrients into synovial fluid. It also helps us access our healing-regeneration system.

By releasing endorphins in the brain, for instance, aerobic exercise transforms depression into an upbeat mood that lasts all day and reduces the need for pain-killing or antidepressant drugs. Because it requires us to act physically, it turns on our enabling effect. In turn, our entire healing-regeneration system then goes to work to help relieve arthritis on every level of the body-mind.

The Fat-Destroying Power of Rhythmic Exercise

Part of the healing effect of aerobic exercise is to elevate the metabolism and burn off surplus body fat. Excess body fat is the number one cause of OA.

For every 3,500 calories expended in aerobic exercise, 1 pound of body fat is lost. In order to lose 1 pound in 10 days, we need only expend 350 calories more per day in exercise than we consume in our diet. The table below shows the approximate number of calories expended per hour by a person weighing 150 pounds while performing various types of low-impact aerobic exercise.

Calories Burned per Hour by Low-Impact Aerobic Exercises

Rowing machine, moderate pace	325
Brisk walking at 4 mph	345
Bicycling at 12 mph	500
Swimming at 1 mph	535
Rowing machine, vigorous pace	650
Stair-climbing machine, vigorous workout	675

Assuming you weigh 150 pounds, 1 hour a day spent swimming, pedalling a stationary bicycle or walking briskly should easily knock a pound off your weight in 10 days. Or an hour a day spent exercising at a more vigorous pace could burn off a pound in a single week.

Extensive research at the Jean Mayer Human Nutrition Research Center at Tufts University has revealed that people become overweight in two ways. First, by consuming too much fat and too many calories in the diet. Second, by becoming sedentary and giving up all exercise. We'll deal with the high-fat diet in Arthritis Fighters #9 and #10.

Boost Your Metabolism with Exercise

Meanwhile, if you're really sincere about beating OA or gout, it's vital to realize right now that *we put on weight because our metabolism slows down when we stop exercising.*

It wasn't until the early 1990s that researchers at Tufts discovered that the biological cause of most corpulence is loss of lean muscle mass due to lack of exercise. Lean muscle mass is another term for our skeletal muscles, that is, the muscles that power every joint in the body. When our muscles become weak and flabby from lack of use, they atrophy and our metabolism plummets. Studies show that from age 30 on, the average sedentary American loses more than 6 pounds of lean muscle mass per decade while gaining 10 pounds of fat.

Unlike fat, muscle is biologically active, meaning it continues to burn calories 24 hours a day, even when we're resting or asleep. The larger our lean muscle mass, the more calories our muscles burn and the higher our metabolism rises.

The best way to restore our lean muscle mass is by strength-building exercises (see AF#7). The next best way is through regular aerobic exercise. Aerobic exercise doesn't build muscles quite as large or as strong as strength-building exercise does. But aerobic exercise *will* restore much of the muscle we have lost. At the same time, the exercise itself burns off several hundred calories of surplus fat per hour.

Don't Cheat Yourself Out of Nature's Best Pain Reliever

The Arthritis Foundation recommends brisk walking for both RA and OA, provided it can be done without discomfort. They suggest beginning with a daily walk of 20 minutes and gradually increasing speed and distance.

Surveys show that 60 percent of people with arthritis walk for exercise and for freedom from stiffness and pain. Some walk 3 to 5 miles every day. In addition to exercising aerobically, others use strength-training machines to build up strength in their knee and thigh muscles. Incredibly, I discovered that some of these people, both men and women, have eventually been able to hike long distances in the mountains.

As one 80-year-old woman recently put it: "Don't cheat yourself out of one of nature's best arthritis pain relievers." This woman had suffered from RA for years. Her flare-ups had ceased, but unless she walked regularly, she still experienced pain in her knees. Four times a week she drove to a nearby shopping mall and walked briskly for 2 hours with members of a local walking club. "If I stopped walking, my joints would stiffen up and the pain would return," she told me.

A small study of 11 women with RA at the University of Michigan confirmed that aerobic exercise brings both physical and psychological benefits. After exercising regularly for 13 weeks on a stationary bicycle, all the women reported increased physical strength and ability to do housework. They also experienced a more optimistic mood, less joint pain and increased pain tolerance. A similar control group experienced none of these benefits. Such results confirm those of many similar studies showing that men and women with either OA or RA almost invariably experience benefits to both body and mind from performing aerobic exercise.

How to Get Started

Consult your doctor and obtain his or her approval before beginning to exercise. It's important to note, however, that some doctors warn their arthritis patients against aerobic exercise because they fear it may be too strenuous. While this may occasionally be true, it is not for most people. So if your doctor has this mistaken view, you may have to switch to a physician who is more in tune with today's fitness culture.

It's best to avoid high-impact aerobic exercises such as jogging, stepping, aerobic dancing or rope skipping. Start out instead with gentle, low-impact exercises like walking, bicycling, swimming or rowing. Stair climbing on a machine may be another option.

Start by doing what is comfortable for you. Then increase gradually. Never push yourself to the point of pain. Once you can walk briskly, swing your arms to increase the cardio-vascular benefit.

Wear the Right Shoes

Anyone with arthritis should wear a well-cushioned pair of athletic fitness walking shoes for aerobic walking. Don't even *think* about walking in cheap jogging or tennis shoes or in shoes with thin soles. Even so, walking shoes needn't cost a fortune. Nowadays top-of-the-line shoes sold in discount stores usually have quite adequate cushioning. While shoes specifically built for walking are obviously best, well-cushioned jogging shoes are almost as good. Shoes that lace up are preferable to shoes with Velcro straps.

Any shoe you buy should have a wide toe box, with enough room to curl your toes and for your big toe to lie flat. Make sure that the shoe grasps your heel firmly but there's still room to insert your forefinger between your heel and the heel of the shoe. The shoe should also be wide enough to allow for some expansion in your feet after you begin to walk. For this reason I suggest you walk briskly for 30 minutes to allow your feet to swell before shopping for a pair of shoes. Also shop in the late afternoon after your feet have swollen to maximum size. Wear the same socks you will wear when walking.

If you have OA or RA of the hips, knees, ankles or spine, try to walk on soft ground. A walking or running track or a grassy trail may be easier on your joints than walking on concrete.

People with arthritis often have foot problems caused by

ill-fitting shoes. A pain in the ball of your foot may be a sign that you need an orthotic. An orthotic is a full or partial support that fits inside your shoe and supports your arch and heel. Often, an over-the-counter arch or heel support sold in drug or shoe stores will relieve any discomfort in your feet while walking.

If that doesn't help, I suggest consulting a podiatrist (an M.D. who specializes in foot disorders) who can custom-design a pair of orthotics. Professionally made orthotics can often work wonders to correct any imbalance in walking caused by arthritis.

Pain Relief May Be Just a Walk Away

Endorphins are the brain's natural pain-killers. Chemically similar to morphine or heroin, these complex peptide molecules bind on to pain receptors in the brain and block out all or most sensations of arthritis pain. Once endorphin release occurs, it takes only a few minutes for all feelings of depression, anxiety and hopelessness to be replaced by strongly positive feelings of optimism, hope and cheerfulness. If you've ever experienced "runner's high," you'll know exactly what I mean.

However, you don't have to run to release the brain's natural narcotics. Unlike pharmaceutical morphine, endorphins are available free of charge to anyone able to exercise aerobically.

All you need do is exercise briskly for 35 minutes at a pace fast enough to elevate the rate of both your pulse and your respiration. When this occurs, the brain begins to release clouds of endorphin. To reach this stage, you may have to speed up your pace a bit so that mild perspiration appears on your brow—except while swimming.

Thousands of people with arthritis take a brisk walk, swim or bike ride first thing in the morning because it makes them feel good for the rest of the day. Once we fall asleep, the endorphins disappear. But we can always get them back by exercising again the following day.

Can Aerobic Exercise Rebuild Damaged Cartilage?

The view of mainstream medicine is that exercise is essential to keep a joint mobile, maintain range of motion and prevent pain and further deterioration. But medical science has yet to prove that any type of exercise has the ability to heal and rebuild damaged cartilage.

However, back in 1986, John H. Bland, a rheumatologist at the University of Vermont, developed a technique that he believed would improve the ability of cartilage cells to reproduce themselves. Bland thought that damaged cartilage might heal and that aerobic exercise might promote that healing.

Although Bland's theory is considered controversial today, substantial evidence exists to support it. For instance, the cells of cartilage are known as "chondrocytes" and they exist in a matrix of gel laced with fiber. When weight is placed on cartilage in a joint, it compresses like a sponge and squeezes waste products out into the synovial fluid to be carried away by lymph and blood. When a joint is at rest, cartilage expands and absorbs synovial fluid. This fluid contains nutrients that are essential to the health and well-being of the chondrocytes.

Bland's claim was that exercise, such as walking, helps this pumping action by alternately compressing and then expanding cartilage in weight-bearing joints. For best results, he suggested walking several times daily for 15 to 20 minutes to create nutrient exchange, then resting for an hour or so. By repeating this cycle several times each day, toxins are expelled from joint cartilage and replaced with healing nutrients.

By walking for short periods several times each day, nutrient exchange is increased to the point where cartilage cells may reproduce themselves and gradually repair the damage done by OA.

Use Your Inner Healing Powers to Boost Exercise Benefits

One thing Bland apparently didn't try was to boost results by incorporating the help of the body's healing-regeneration system. As you may recall from Chapter 2, provided you believe in and have faith in a method; understand exactly how it works and are willing to use your mind and muscles to do what it takes to succeed, your body's healing-regeneration system may increase your chances of success by 70 percent.

For example, if Bland's method works 10 percent of the time, then your inner healing powers may raise your chances of success to 17 percent or more. If you haven't read Chapter 2 or don't remember it, I suggest going back and absorbing it thoroughly before you try this, or any other, action-step.

One criticism leveled at Bland's method is that in a joint afflicted with OA, nodules of cartilage called "osteophytes" may form and then break off and intefere with joint motion. Nonetheless, if you have the needed time and are really serious about recovering from OA—and if you're willing to tap into your body's inner healing powers as well—then this method may well be worth a try.

The technique works best on knee cartilage damaged by OA. If you can't walk, pedalling a bicycle works almost as well. Remember that your doctor's approval is essential before you try this method. And for maximum benefit, you should continue to exercise aerobically for the rest of your life. Otherwise, your cartilage could begin to deteriorate once more.

Exercise Aerobically If You're Unable to Walk

Whenever possible, I recommend walking outdoors in daylight. Being outdoors in natural light prevents depression and elevates your mood. But if you can't exercise outdoors, then walk in a mall, on an indoor track or on a treadmill in a gym or at home. Or consider one of the four optional ways of exercising aerobically described below.

- *Stairclimbers.* If for some reason the impact of walking bothers your feet, consider exercising on a stairclimbing machine. Most gyms have at least one stairclimber nowadays, and they're becoming increasingly popular with orthopedic surgeons for rehabilitating knees after surgery.

  Essentially, you place each foot on a pedal and step up and down alternately with much the same motion you'd use to climb real stairs. But a stairclimber is impact-free, and it allows you to "climb" stairs without having to walk back down again. Walking downstairs is far more stressful to joints than walking up.

  Begin by taking shallow steps and deepen them gradually as your leg muscles gain strength. There's one important caution: Anyone with arthritis should use a stairclimber only under the supervision of a physical therapist or physician.

- *Bicycling.* Bicycling benefits most cases of arthritis in the knee or hip, though, occasionally, pedaling may worsen inflammation and swelling. Riding outdoors on

143

a real bicycle is far more interesting than riding a stationary bicycle indoors. But most people with arthritis lack the skill, or the opportunity, to ride a real bicycle.

On a stationary bicycle, set the resistance to "low" to begin and increase gradually. Also adjust the seat to allow your leg to almost, but not quite, straighten as the pedal reaches its lowest point.

In gyms, avoid bicycles programmed to stiffen resistance every few minutes to resemble riding uphill. On a real bike, you'd shift down the gears to ease the strain of pedaling uphill. But gears don't exist on a stationary bike and a programmed ride could create knee problems for a person with arthritis.

- *Swimming.* Swimming is an excellent aerobic exercise that places zero impact on joints, but it could conceivably stress the shoulders, elbows or wrists. So ease off if you feel any pain in your shoulders.

  For anyone with arthritis, the pool temperature should range between 80° and 84°F. Some 25-meter training pools are kept at a cooler temperature for serious swimmers and a temperature under 80°F could possibly worsen arthritis pain.

  If you're unable to swim, try walking along the pool bottom in waist-deep water, using your hands as paddles. Try walking backwards as well as forwards.

- *Rowing.* Rowing a real boat using oars, or using a rowing machine, is a splendid way to restore strength and mobility to the upper body. To provide whole-body exercise, most rowing machines and racing shells feature a sliding seat powered by flexing the knees.

  However, you can row perfectly well, and give your body a splendid aerobic workout, by bending from the hips instead of using a sliding seat. Dories, skiffs and similar traditional rowboats can all be rowed without a sliding seat. In a gym, other machines can provide the motions of rowing so you don't have to flex your knees at all. Begin with about 10 minutes a day and increase gradually to 35 minutes or more.

ARTHRITIS FIGHTER #6: Let Good Posture Help You Beat Arthritis Pain

---

Many people with arthritis unknowingly worsen their pain through poor posture. Poor body alignment often contributes to deformities of the hips, ankles, knees and spine by placing unnecessary and unnatural stress on muscles and joints.

But this need never happen.

You can help beat arthritis by maintaining correct posture when you stand, walk, sit, bend, lift or lie down. Years ago, pioneers of the modern body-mind movement such as F. M. Alexander and Moshe Feldenkrais developed exciting new theories of postural balance through which anyone can learn to move every joint with fluid ease.

For instance, Alexander discovered that we could minimize stress on our muscles and joints by leading off all movements with the head. Try it for yourself and you'll immediately feel your spine stretching out and the rest of your body following with graceful ease.

Next time you get up from a chair, let your head lead the way while the rest of your body follows. It's more an attitude than anything else, which is why physiotherapists call it the "body-mind movement. "But it's a proven fact. Whenever you visualize yourself in your mind moving lightly and effortlessly and without stiffness or pain, then your body will immediately begin to move in that way.

145

You'll find it easy enough to visualize your head leading your body upwards. But with a little practice, you'll find it equally easy to let your head lead your movements when you sit down or walk downstairs.

Lack of space prevents going into more detail here about the wonderful movement systems developed by Alexander and Feldenkrais. Yet almost every library has illustrated books describing their methods. Besides defusing arthritis pain and stiffness, both men discovered that the way we move our bodies changes the way we see ourselves and view the world.

Tips You Can Begin Using Immediately to Improve Your Posture

People with arthritis frequently adopt a swayback posture that substantially increases risk of lower back pain. To avoid this risk—whether sitting or standing—try to maintain an erect posture. Keep your spine straight. Avoid slouching or hunching over. Sit only in upright chairs. And never sit or stand in one position for longer than 30 minutes. Otherwise, your knees, back, neck, shoulders, wrists and fingers will become stiff and sore.

To begin standing erect, simply relax and drop your shoulders and tilt back the top of your pelvis. This immediately flattens the abdomen and tucks in the buttocks.

Never try to adopt a military stance. But do keep your head straight and in line with your spine. Pull your shoulders back. Raise your chest. And avoid slumping as you walk. Balance your weight equally on both feet when standing and keep them 6 to 8 inches apart and parallel or slightly turned out. Knees should be straight but not locked.

If you *must* stand for longer than 30 minutes, relieve the

stress on your joints by raising one foot on a low box or stool so that the hip and knee are flexed. Change sides frequently.

Since your body carries out whatever blueprint you visualize for it in your mind, imagine yourself suspended from a hook by the top of your head. Picture your whole body hanging loose and relaxed like a puppet but with your spine straight and your whole body erect. I often visualize myself this way when I'm walking and I can feel my entire body respond immediately.

Take Years off Your Appearance by Sitting Correctly

Slouching in a deep, stuffed chair or on a couch for hours at a time stresses the spine and invariably worsens arthritis pain. Instead, sit only in a straight-backed chair. Place your buttocks all the way back and sit upright with your feet flat on the floor. A straight-backed chair provides firm support for the lower back, where most stress occurs. By sitting upright, you also rest as much of your thighs as possible on the chair seat. If you start to feel uncomfortable after 20 to 30 minutes, don't slouch down. Get up and walk around for a few minutes.

If you must sit for longer than 30 minutes, use a chair with armrests and place your feet on a box or stool so that your knees are higher than your hips. The armrests should be high enough to prevent any tendency to hunch.

When working at a desk, be sure to sit erect and keep your shoulders relaxed. Your elbows should be at right angles to your body when typing.

For sleeping, a firm mattress and a single pillow (or two if they are thin) are best. Lie on your side, if possible, and use the pillow to keep your head in line with your spine. A contour foam pillow may help with this. If you're like most

147

people, you'll wake up briefly once every 90 minutes during the night. At that point, which marks the end of a sleep cycle, turn over if you can and lie on your other side through the next sleep cycle. Change position after each sleep cycle to avoid stiffness.

Always lift a heavy weight by bending your knees and keeping your back straight. Always use your legs to raise or lower your body. Try to distribute the weight over as many joints and muscles as possible. For example, grasp the weight with both arms instead of only one.

By upgrading their posture, some people with arthritis report they have reduced their pain by at least 33 percent. You can do even better when you also restore your muscle strength as described in the following Arthritis Fighter.

ARTHRITIS FIGHTER #7: Let Your Muscles Ease the Agony of Arthritis

---

A torrent of new scientific discoveries in recent years has clearly identified weak skeletal muscles as the physical cause of most cases of OA and of some cases of RA as well.

It works like this. Metabolism is the chemical process in the body that releases energy from food. Key to our basic metabolic rate is the size and weight of our skeletal muscles (called by physiologists our "lean muscle mass.") This is because body muscle is biologically active. Even when at rest or while we're asleep, our muscles continue to burn surplus calories that otherwise would turn into body fat. The more muscle we possess, the higher it turns up our metabolism and the faster we burn up our reserves of stored fat.

Body fat, by comparison, is biologically inactive and burns almost zero calories. We put on weight because a fat-laden diet fills the body with surplus calories while an inactive, sedentary lifestyle allows our muscles to atrophy and become flabby and weak.

As our muscles fade, our metabolism plunges. Fat bulges out where muscle once kept the body slender and trim. Today, one-third of all Americans are seriously overweight. Every extra pound of fat we add places extra stress on the joints in our spine, hips, knees, ankles and feet. Gradually, this excess body weight wears down the cartilage in our weight-bearing joints. In as few as 10 years, an obese man or woman can develop a severe case of OA.

Now Here's the Rest of the Story

Healthy cartilage acts as a natural shock-absorber. When we walk, run or jump, it cushions our knees from the shock of each impact. Strong muscles work as additional shock absorbers.

But when cartilage wears thin, as in OA, and muscles shrink from lack of use, nothing is left to cushion the shock of impact in our weight-bearing joints.

Thus far, no one has come up with a really dependable way to repair damaged cartilage. *But we can rebuild our muscles.* And strong muscles *can* replace much of the shock-absorbing function that is destroyed by OA.

To make it even clearer: Increasing our lean muscle mass through strength-building exercises can do more to fight arthritis than almost any other single step.

1. It can burn away surplus body fat, which is a major cause of both OA and RA.

2. When cartilage in weight-bearing joints is damaged by

OA or RA, strong muscles can take over and act as shock absorbers in place of damaged cartilage.

3. Since muscle weakness can affect the alignment and function of a joint, it's essential to use strength training, if possible, to maintain muscle tone. Strong muscles also help a person walk well.

4. Weak abdominal and back muscles are largely responsible for lower back pain, a common form of arthritis. By restoring these muscles to their original size and strength, and by using the stretching exercises in AF#4, most cases of lower back pain can be permanently eliminated.

The One Best Strategy for Beating Arthritis

I can't overemphasize the fact that by rebuilding our muscles, we can overcome much of the pain and stiffness of OA, knee pain, lower back pain and, in some cases, of RA as well. And we can do it in just a few weeks or months, regardless of gender or age.

A few years ago, researchers in Finland found that when people with knee pain did exercises to strengthen the quadricep muscles in their thighs, 70 percent experienced complete recovery.

Few of us are ever too old to benefit from strength-training exercise. Several years ago, Dr. Maria Fiatarone studied a group of 63 women and 37 men aged 72 to 98 at Boston's Hebrew Rehab Center for the Aged. Their average age was 87 and one-third were over 90. One-third of the group worked out regularly on strength-training machines, one-third took nutritional supplements and one-third did nothing. After a few weeks, all the strength-training group had increased their muscle strength, muscle size, walking speed and stair-climbing ability. They also displayed powerful psychological benefits including heightened self-image, increased confidence and optimism and a greatly increased quality of life. Nutritional supplements alone produced no increase in strength or mobility.

This, and several similar studies, prove that regardless of age, or of how atrophied a person's muscles may be, both strength and muscle mass can be improved as well as mobility, balance and endurance.

How to Send Your Metabolism Soaring

Nor does strength-training benefit only men. In another study by HNRC, 40 women aged 50 to 70 were divided into two groups. One group performed five different strength-training exercises twice a week. The control group did nothing. One year later, the women in the strength-training group had lost an average of 3 to 4 pounds of fat and gained 4 pounds of muscle. They also increased bone mass in the hip and spine and had an improved sense of balance. All these factors worsened in the control group.

Losing 4 pounds of fat may not sound like a lot, but gaining 4 pounds of muscle is enough to send a person's metabolism soaring. As the months went by, most of the women in the strength-training group began to enjoy their exercise workouts. Almost all began to lead more active lives and several took up dancing.

How to Calculate Your Personal Metabolism

Until very recently, calculating your personal metabolism was difficult and expensive. But with the aid of a pocket calculator, a new, simple formula allows almost anyone to calculate his or her personal metabolism in a couple of minutes.

Your resting metabolism is the number of calories your

body-mind consumes each 24 hours while completely at rest. Eat fewer calories than your metabolism and you lose weight. Eat more and you gain.

MEN

Step 1. Multiply your height in inches by 12.7.
Step 2. Multiply your weight in pounds by 6.3.
Step 3. Combine these two numbers and add 66.
Step 4. Multiply your age by 6.8.
Step 5. Subtract the result of step 4 from step 3.
The result is your resting rate of metabolism.

WOMEN

Step 1. Multiply your height in inches by 4.7.
Step 2. Multiply your weight in pounds by 4.3.
Step 3. Combine these numbers and add 655.
Step 4. Multiply your age by 4.7.
Step 5. Subtract the result of step 4 from step 3.
The result is your resting rate of metabolism.

Naturally, your resting metabolism completely excludes the effect of exercise. By recalculating your metabolism once each month, you can easily keep track of any increase in your resting metabolic rate.

What Exactly Is Strength Training?

As you work out with free weights or strength-building machines, strength training (also called weight training, strength building, resistance training, progressive resistance training or

152

isotonics) increases lean muscle mass. The weights or resistance used are much lighter than those needed for body building, and no one expects you to become Ms. or Mr. Universe.

But doesn't aerobic exercise build and strengthen muscles, you may ask? Certainly, brisk walking, bicycling or swimming exercises muscles and strengthens them to some extent (see AF#5). But to really increase your lean muscle mass to where it can start burning off weight, and cushioning your knees and other joints, you have to pump iron.

Don't let that term put you off.

Nowadays, it's mostly weight lifters and body builders who use free weights—that is, meaning barbells and dumbbells. Most strength training is done on machines in a gym or spa. The concept of "no pain, no gain" is out these days. You can begin with very light weights and increase resistance in easy, comfortable stages.

For a modest monthly fee, a typical gym will let you work out as often as you like, and most gyms have treadmills, stairclimbers, stationary bikes, free weights and classes in aerobics, stretching and yoga. Larger gyms often have a swimming pool and an indoor track as well.

If you live far from a gym, you can buy a set of free weights with a bench and stand. If your goal is to increase lean muscle mass all over your body—in order to raise your metabolism and shed surplus pounds—free weights are just as effective as strength-training machines.

Why Strength-Training Machines May Be Better Than Weights

However, free weights may not be the best answer for anyone with arthritis. This is because it's almost essential to have a machine for exercising the thigh muscles that cushion the knees. So if you plan to exercise at home, I recommend investing in a good quality multistation gym machine. Besides allowing you to do leg curls and knee extenders for strengthening muscles in the thighs, these machines let you build up almost every other muscle group in the body. (Be sure that any machine you buy allows you to do leg curls and knee-extender exercises.)

However, most people find it faster, cheaper and more convenient to work out on machines in a gym. The machines are of top quality, and each is specifically designed to strengthen an isolated muscle group. You can hire a fitness instructor to prepare a custom-tailored workout schedule and guide you through several initial sessions while you learn to use the equipment.

Compared with free weights, which must be taken on and off a barbell, all it takes to ready a machine for use is to insert a pin in a slot. Machines also reduce any risk of injury.

Women Need Strength Training More Than Men

Some women may hesitate to sign up for a strength-training session in a gym. Nowadays, however, working out on strength-building machines is no longer exclusively for males. All over America, women are realizing that lack of muscular exertion is the reason why their bodies age, and they're rethinking and redefining their relationship to strength-building exercise. In the typical spa or gym, one-third of the people using resistance-training equipment are likely to be women.

Don't worry about building large, bulky muscles. It's next to impossible for a woman to build muscles as large as a man's. If you still feel that strength building is unfeminine, then have a fitness instructor show you around a local spa or gym. Chances are, you'll see women of all ages, shapes and sizes working out on strength-training machines.

Lack of space prevents me from describing how to do specific strength-training exercises. Instead, my purpose is to guide you toward starting a regular strength-building exercise program that focuses on helping you beat arthritis. Every library has a selection of books on strength training, while fitness instructors are available at almost every spa or gym to help you get started.

Actually, you can begin a strength-training program without weights or machines by using either calisthenics or isometric exercises or both. You'll find several helpful exercises described below, and you can start using them almost immediately.

As with any other exercise, it's essential to have your doctor's permission before you begin. No one with arthritis, or with any other disease, disorder or dysfunction, should attempt to use strength-building exercises without medical approval. Assuming you have that, the following guidelines will introduce you to strength training and how to get started.

How to Rebuild Your Lean Muscle Mass

The following nine steps will help you rebuild your lean muscle mass.

1. A repetition (rep) is one complete exercise movement such as raising a weight and lowering it back down to the starting position. A set is a series of consecutive reps, typically 8 reps, and "1-RM" is the maximum weight you can lift at one time in a single rep. If you can do another rep immediately, that's not 1-RM. You must increase the weight until you can do just one rep and no more. It's important to

determine your 1-RM for each exercise you plan to do. Knowing your 1-RM tells you how much weight to use.

2. To increase strength, you must lift about 80 percent of your 1-RM. For example, if your 1-RM for a certain exercise is 100 pounds, start at 80 pounds. At this level, you should be able to do 6 to 8 reps. To make it easier, start off at 70 percent of 1-RM. Then work up gradually to where you're using 80 percent. Working out with lighter weights, or with less resistance, is fine to get started. But to really build up your lean muscle mass, you need to lift at 80 percent of your 1-RM level.

3. Do no more than 8 to 9 reps in each set. If you're able to do 10 or more, it's time to increase the weight. However, it's acceptable to do only 3, 4 or 5 reps in a set. The greater the resistance, or the heavier the weight, the more muscle cells you will break down and the larger and stronger your muscle will become. Perform 3 sets of each exercise on your workout program, making sure to pause for 1 to 2 seconds between each rep in a set. You can then rest for 1 to 1½ minutes between sets and for 1 to 2 minutes before starting a new exercise. Most exercisers walk slowly up and down or stretch out their muscles during these rests.

4. Increase resistance as you build strength so that you push your muscles to the limit of their capacity while performing a set. As your workouts progress and you gain strength, this will become increasingly easy. Try to avoid going all the way to complete muscle fatigue. Should your muscles fail before completing the final rep, reduce the resistance or weight by one step and immediately do several more reps. Fitness trainers call this "breakdown training." The extra reps fatigue additional muscle fibers and these grow back swiftly into larger, stronger muscles. But breakdown training works only if your muscles fail and you do the additional reps immediately. This is possible only with a machine and if you're in reasonably good condition.

5. Avoid holding your breath while performing strength-building exercises. Each exercise has two phases. The *concentric* phase occurs as you use maximum exertion to contract a set of muscles as you lift a weight; always exhale during the concentric phase. The *eccentric* phase occurs as you slowly lower the weight and return to your starting position; always inhale during the eccentric phase.

6. Perform each movement at a slow-to-moderate pace, taking 6 to 10 seconds for each rep. This ensures that you exercise only the target muscles. Working out more rapidly creates momentum which brings other muscles into play. Always move slowly during the eccentric phase and feel resistance as you lower the weight. Much of your new muscle mass is built during this phase.

Mild muscle pain after a workout often indicates that your body is building new muscle. Wait until the discomfort has gone before working out again—usually 2 to 3 days. To give your muscles an opportunity to rebuild and grow, schedule strength-building exercise on alternate days. During the rest days in between, you can still do aerobic or stretching exercises.

7. To restore lean muscle mass over your entire body, focus on exercises that increase strength in these muscle groups:

abdominals   pectorals
lower back   quadriceps
upper back   shoulders
hamstrings   triceps
biceps

You need only one exercise for each muscle group, making a total of nine exercises . Begin by doing a single set, then add a second or third. Your muscles should feel tired by the ninth rep in each set. If you can do a tenth rep, raise the weight or resistance to the next step. You should easily complete 3 sets of these 9 exercises in well under an hour using machines. With free weights, it will take a few minutes more. Performed every second day, a program like this should give you a significant increase in lean muscle mass in 8 weeks or so.

8. Avoid working out on an empty stomach. Eat a small high-energy meal of whole grains or bread, starchy vegetables and beans or sunflower seeds and raisins about an hour before starting to exercise. If you eat a full meal, allow 2 hours to elapse. After a light, high-energy snack you need wait only 30 minutes. Take a sports drink, a glass of water or a cup of herbal, black or green tea 30 to 60 minutes before starting. And drink as much as you like.

Wear loose-fitting clothing or exercise tights. Before starting any strength-training workout, it's especially essential to warm up by walking as briskly as you can, swinging your arms for a few minutes and then doing a few brief stretches.

9. When muscles that support arthritic joints are seldom used, they frequently atrophy, becoming smaller and weaker. This provides less support to the very joints that need the most support. When doing exercises to strengthen these muscles, focus on strengthening *all* the muscles around a joint, not merely one group. For example, for the knee, you should strengthen both the quadriceps muscles on the front of the thigh and the hamstrings on the back of the thigh. Otherwise, if these muscle groups are unbalanced, they can create a misalignment in the knee joint or in the kneecap that worsens arthritis instead of improving it. Strengthening both muscle groups in the thigh helps protect the knee against the impact of walking.

Here is how to do several strength-building exercises that benefit arthritis.

To Prevent Lower Back Pain

If you have access to a gym, you can build up your abdominal muscles (abs) by working out on a crunch-up machine, a Roman Chair or a sit-up slant board. Otherwise, try the three exercises below.

THE SIMPLE CRUNCH-UP

Directly or indirectly, most cases of lower back pain are due to weak, flabby *rectus abdominis* (ab) muscles that run up the middle of the abdomen. Instead of the traditional sit-up, which may lead to even more back pain, most fitness instructors today build up the abs with an exercise called the simple crunch-up.

Step 1. Lie on your back on a rug on the floor with your feet next to a couch or chair.

Step 2. Raise your lower legs and feet and place them on the chair or couch so that your knees and hips are both bent 90 degrees. Your buttocks and back remain on the floor.

Step 3. Fold your arms across your chest.

Step 4. Pull in your chin to your chest. Then, raise your head, neck and shoulders off the floor and lift them as high as you can, tightening your abs. Keep your lower back pressed against the floor. Raise your head and shoulders slowly, taking about a second to reach the top of the crunch. Exhale throughout this movement.

Step 5. Hold the crunch for one full second, then slowly lower your head, neck and shoulders back down. This eccentric phase should take 2 seconds and you should inhale while doing it. Take care not to lower your shoulders all the way back to the floor.

Step 6. Just before your shoulders touch the floor, and while you still have full tension in your abs, repeat Step 4 and begin to raise your head, neck and shoulders in a second crunch-up. Then repeat Step 5, lowering your shoulders almost back down to the floor.

Step 7. Without ever lowering your shoulders all the way back to the floor, repeat the crunch-ups as many times as possible. When your abs fatigue, lie back down on the floor. This counts as one set. Most people can do 8 reps of the crunch-up in their first set.

Keep all movements slow and controlled, especially the eccentric phase as you lower back down. This is when most of the strength building occurs. Avoid building up any momentum or you may develop your back muscles more than your abs.

Do 3 sets of 8 reps each, if you can. As your strength increases, gradually increase the number of reps in each set to 25. When you can do that, begin to hold the top of the crunch for 2 seconds, then for 3 and finally for 4 seconds. When you can do that, take 2 seconds to raise up and 3 to 4 seconds to lower back down.

Maintain tension on your abs the whole time you are doing a set, and be sure to avoid lowering your shoulders all the way back down to the floor until you have completed a full set.

THE ADVANCED CRUNCH-UP

While the simple crunch-up strengthens the *rectus abdominis*, it does little for the internal and external obliques, the muscles at the sides of the trunk. These muscles also play a key role in preventing lower back pain. You can easily strengthen the obliques by using an exercise physiologists call the advanced crunch-up.

Step 1. Lie on your back on a rug on the floor with your feet flat on the floor and knees flexed.

Step 2. Drop both your knees to the right as far as you can.

Step 3. Place your left hand beneath your head and your right hand under your right thigh. As you hold this position, perform as many crunch-ups as you can in exactly the same way as when you did the simple crunch-up. Again avoid lowering your shoulders all the way back to the floor until you have completed a set.

Step 4. When you have completed a set, switch the position of your hands so that your right hand is behind your head and your left hand is under your left thigh. Lower your knees all the way to the left. Do another set while holding this position.

Complete up to 3 sets on each side, swapping the position of your hands after each set. As you gain strength, increase the number of reps in each set up to a maximum of 25. Then increase the length of time you hold each position, just as you did for the simple crunch-up.

Strengthening the Abs with Leg Lowering

Raising the legs has been a popular abs strengthener for decades. It has also aggravated innumerable cases of lower back pain. In recent years, exercise physiologists have discovered that almost all strength-building benefits occur during the eccentric phase as the legs are being lowered. They have also found that most injuries occur during the concentric phase as both legs are being raised together.

A new version, known as "leg lowering"—raising each leg separately, then slowly lowering both legs together—provides all the benefits of the original exercise while eliminating almost all the drawbacks.

Step 1. Lie on your back on a rug on the floor with your knees straight and your legs fully extended and close together.

Step 2. Raise one leg to a 45-degree angle. Hold it there while you raise the other leg to the same position. Hold both legs in the air for a few seconds.

Step 3. Keeping your legs together, lower them as slowly as possible back to the floor. Breathe normally throughout. Take a brief rest, then repeat this exercise up to 10 times. This counts as a set.

To Prevent Osteoarthritis in the Knees

The knee is a fragile joint that depends on the quadricep and hamstring muscles in the thigh for much of its support. When one of these muscles is stronger than the other, the resulting imbalance can worsen cartilage damage in the knee joint and in the kneecap. The simple exercises below help to restore strength and balance to knee muscles so that they provide support and shock absorption to the knee.

THE KNEE EXTENDER EXERCISE

The best way to strengthen the quadricep muscles in the front of the thigh is to use a knee-extender machine in a gym. Virtually all gyms and spas have these machines nowadays. Basically, you sit on a seat and raise your lower leg and foot until it is straight at the knee and stretched out in front of you. To build strength, however, you must raise your leg against resistance. So, in practice, you won't be able to fully straighten your knee.

Most machines allow you to extend one leg at a time, or you can double the resistance and extend both legs together. For anyone with arthritis, I suggest exercising one leg at a time. This permits you to select a resistance against which you can raise your leg about 70 degrees. Be sure to raise your leg and foot slowly, hold, then slowly lower your leg and foot back down again.

Do as many reps as you can up to a maximum of 10. When you can do 11, use a heavier weight. Exercise both knees equally, even though only one may be painful. As you gain strength, progress to doing 3 sets with each knee. You may experience mild pain for a few minutes after using a knee-extender machine. Stop immediately if you feel a severe or persistent pain and do not continue this exercise.

If you don't have access to a knee-extender machine, you can do this exercise at home. Sit on an upright chair with both feet flat on the floor. Raise one foot so that your leg is straight at the knee and stretched out in front of you. Lower it back to the floor. This is the motion you need.

Next, place a light weight (1 or 2 pounds) on your foot, such as a sandbag or a foot or ankle weight, and repeat the exercise up to 10 times. Continue to exercise as described for the knee-extender machine, taking care not to fully extend the knee to the point where your leg is totally straight.

The problem with ankle weights is that your quads will soon become so strong that you must use extremely heavy weights on your ankle or foot. When you reach that stage, you might consider investing in a multistation gym machine or possibly a knee machine.

THE STANDING CALF RAISE EXERCISE

Rising up and down on the ball of your foot strengthens the calf muscle. This powerful muscle supports the ankle and helps to cushion the knee from below. In a gym, look for a machine that is usually called the Standing Calf. This machine lets you place the balls of both feet on a low step while your shoulders go under a padded yoke linked to a series of weights. Using your calf muscles, you gently rise up on the balls of your feet, lifting the yoke linked to the weights. Then you slowly lower your heels all the way down. Select a weight that allows you to perform about 8 reps to a set.

If you don't have access to a Standing Calf machine, try this. Place a piece of 2"-by-4" lumber, or a thick book or a brick, flat on the floor so that it forms a step about 2 inches high. Hold on to the wall or a doorpost or chair. Place the balls of both feet on the step, with your heels on the floor. Then slowly raise your heels as high as you can, hold and, just as slowly, lower your heels back down to the floor.

As you gain strength and flexibility, do the exercise using only one foot. When that becomes easy, raise the height of the step another inch. You can increase resistance even more by performing the exercise at a still slower pace.

PARTIAL SQUAT

Requiring no equipment, this exercise is a splendid way to strengthen your quadriceps muscles. Begin by standing erect with your feet a shoulder width apart. Slowly bend your knees and lower your buttocks about 6 inches, using the same motion as though you were about to sit in a chair. Then slowly raise back up. Practice until you can do 3 sets of 10 reps each.

Since a full squat may cause knee damage, never lower your buttocks more than 6 inches. You can increase resistance by performing this exercise at an ever slower pace.

THE WALL SITTING EXERCISE

Here's another exercise to strengthen the quadriceps. Stand upright with your back against a wall and your feet a shoulder width apart. Keeping your back pressed against the wall, bend your knees so that you slide slowly down the wall until your thighs are parallel to the floor. Hold for as long as you can. Then slowly return to the upright position. Use the palms of your hands to help your body slide up and down the wall. Repeat 3 to 5 times. Do not use this exercise if you have chondromalacia or if you feel any knee pain.

THE LEG CURL EXERCISE

This exercise is best performed on a leg curl machine in a gym. Depending on the machine, you can curl back both legs together or one leg at a time. If you have arthritis, I suggest doing curls with one knee at a time. Select a weight that allows you to do up to 10 reps, and you will quickly build strength in your hamstring muscles at the back of your thigh.

Without a machine, you can use leg weights. Simply stand upright, hold on to something and curl one foot and ankle backwards and upwards as high as you can raise them.

Alternately, try this: Lie on your back on a rug on the floor beside a bed with a fairly stiff mattress. Remove your shoes. Raise and bend your knees and place you feet flat on the bed. Now raise your buttocks and lower back off the floor so that your weight is borne by your shoulders and feet. Keeping this position, raise and lower your buttocks one time. Be sure to use both legs together; note that you can't control the resistance. Each movement is 1 rep. Perform up to 10 reps in a set.

Each time you raise your buttocks up and down you use your hamstrings in essentially the same way as when you use a leg-curl machine. It may take a little practice and you may have to use your elbows at first. But most people find this a worthwhile substitute for the machine.

Another way to strengthen muscles in your lower back is to do the Locust Pose described in AF#4.

To Strengthen Muscles When a Joint Is Inflamed

Pushing hard against an immovable wall is a good way to strengthen muscles without moving an inflamed joint. It's known as "isometric exercising."

To try it, stand in a doorway and place one hand on either side of the doorframe. Then push as hard as you can with both arms. The doorframe shouldn't move. Neither should you or any of your joints. But your muscles were forced to contract and to work hard. You just performed an isometric exercise.

Doing isometrics is a sound way to strengthen muscles without moving a joint. Here are several examples of isometric exercises. Hold each one for 6 seconds. Then relax and repeat as many times as possible up to a maximum of 10.

TO STRENGTHEN ARM AND SHOULDER MUSCLES

Clasp your hands together in front of your chest and press as hard as you can for 6 seconds. Then release. Still holding this position, grasp each wrist with the other hand. Using your shoulder muscles, try to pull your hands apart without letting go. Pull as hard as you can for six seconds. Then release.

TO STRENGTHEN NECK MUSCLES

Exercise A. Place the palm of your left hand against the front of your left temple and the palm of your right hand against the front of the right temple. Push your head forward against the resistance of your arms and hands.

Exercise B. Clasp both hands at the back of your head and pull gently forward while you resist with your neck muscles. Gradually increase the tension.

166

Exercise C. Lie on your back on a rug on the floor with a comfortable cushion or pillow under your head. Press your head back into the pillow as hard as you can and hold for 6 seconds. Then release, and without raising your shoulders, lift your head up off the pillow as high as you can and relax.

The Pros and Cons of Isometric Exercises

These are just a few of several isometric exercises you can do by pitting one set of muscles against another or by pitting your muscles against an immovable object. In each case, you can strengthen your muscles without having to move a joint that may be painful or inflamed.

However, if you have high blood pressure, you should not use isometric exercises without your doctor's approval. And while isometric exercises do strengthen muscles, you should know that isotonic exercises—in which a joint is moved against a resistance—are usually more effective.

When you use exercise to help beat arthritis, you endow yourself with a host of other benefits. Exercising aerobically one day, and doing strength-building exercises the following day, can help everyone look and feel years younger. Together with some yoga stretches, exercising regularly can improve the quality of life of a person with arthritis more than anything else.

In conjunction with a plant-based diet (see AF#10), exercise can dramatically cut your risk of ever developing cancer, heart or renal disease, hypertension and stroke, Type II (adult-onset) diabetes, osteoporosis, emphysema, benign prostate enlargement, obesity and even cataracts or macular degeneration of the retina.

So if you hope to remain healthy and recover from arthritis, exercise is not merely an option. It's an imperative.

CHAPTER SEVEN

The Nutritional Approach: Fight Arthritis with Food and Nutrition

Apart from a grudging admission that rich foods cause gout, mainline medical research generally denies any link between arthritis and food or nutrition. For decades, medical science also denied that heart disease or cancer was caused by diet.

Today we know better. Science has proven that the principal cause of both diseases is the high-fat, low-fiber content of the Standard American Diet. The newest research shows that when we eat fewer foods of animal origin and increasing amounts of fruits, vegetables, whole grains and legumes, we can dramatically lower our risk of developing either of these killer diseases.

While the link between food and arthritis is not as clear, a number of small studies have shown that replacing flesh foods and fat in the diet with more fruits and vegetables very definitely helps recovery from OA, RA and gout. The Arthritis Fighters in this chapter expand on these findings and demonstrate how you can use them as part of a whole-person strategy for overcoming arthritis and gout.

First, a few words of caution. Several studies have shown that fasting almost always relieves the pain and symptoms of RA. No one doubts this. But fasting can be dangerous for anyone with RA and also for people with OA, gout, diabetes and many other diseases and disorders. Fasting produces low blood sugar in everyone, and I recommend that you do *not* use it. It is equally unwise to lose weight for RA or any other autoimmune disease without your physician's approval.

Again, if you have any digestive condition which might be affected by adopting a high-fiber diet, if you have ever had surgery for any digestive tract problem or if you are at risk for any kind of blockage of the gastrointestinal tract, you should consult your doctor before changing to a diet high in grains, fruits, vegetables and legumes.

ARTHRITIS FIGHTER #8: Defeat Osteoarthritis by Peeling Off the Pounds

---

Betty is 45 pounds overweight and has OA in her right knee and hip. Almost every day, Betty has a frustrating time at the office.

Some people might take a prescription tranquilizer. Others might choose to defuse their stress with a brisk walk. But

Betty has a different kind of tranquilizer in mind. She heads for the refrigerator and begins to mindlessly gulp down ice cream. Within minutes, her stomach is filled and she immediately feels better.

But her bathroom scales tell a different story. Week by week Betty's weight is creeping up and the pain in her knee and hip is gradually worsening.

By using food as a tranquilizer, Betty has become seriously overweight. Betty is just one of millions of American men and women who try to eat their way out of stress, unhappiness, loneliness or frustration. All too often they end up, not free of stress, but overweight and feeling the first symptoms of osteoarthritis. For decades, it's been observed that overweight people have a much higher incidence of debilitating OA than people of normal weight.

A classic 16-year study of overweight students at Johns Hopkins Medical School conclusively demonstrated that chubby men—those who carry extra weight in early adulthood—have almost twice the risk of developing OA later in life than men of normal weight.

Twenty pounds of extra weight is all it takes to begin breaking down cartilage in weight-bearing joints. In the John Hopkins study, the heaviest students—those who averaged 190 pounds—were 3.5 times more likely to develop OA in the hip and knee later on than the lightest students, who averaged only 146 pounds.

Shedding Surplus Weight Often Cuts Osteoarthritis Pain

Another recent study at Boston University School of Medicine showed that losing weight—by even a moderate amount—can dramatically lower the risk of ever developing OA. By following 64 women with recently diagnosed OA of the knee and 728 women free of the condition, researchers developed a model showing that a woman 5'11" tall who loses 11 pounds over a 10-year period cuts the risk of developing OA by 50 percent. Women with shorter or heavier bodies can achieve similar protection by losing weight in roughly the same proportion.

The study also showed that, provided your weight does not fall below the ideal level, the more weight you lose, the more you reduce your risk of ever developing OA of the knee. Researchers also concluded that, even if you are already overweight and have OA of the knee, shedding surplus weight may still help relieve pain and minimize further damage.

But excess body weight may not be entirely responsible for OA. Since virtually all overweight people have a high level of body fat, some researchers suspect that chemical or hormonal changes triggered by being fat are what actually damage cartilage in joints.

Indications are that cartilage breaks down only when it is deficient in certain essential nutrients or is being attacked by free radicals. This may explain why losing weight also helps people with OA in their hands.

Being Overweight May Cause Osteoarthritis in the Hands

When researchers from the University of Michigan School of Public Health followed 1,300 residents of Tecumseh, Michigan, for 23 years, they found that people who were 20 percent or more overweight at the start of the study were 3 times more likely to develop OA in their hands than people of the same age with normal weight.

The researchers also found that being overweight frequently precedes OA. They discovered that the degree to which a person is overweight is also the strongest predictor of carpal tunnel syndrome, another form of arthritis.

Being overweight has also been identified as a possible cause of RA. A small Japanese study done in 1993 helps explain why. When the blood of 19 overweight Japanese was analyzed for immune reactions, it was found that obesity can dangerously weaken the response of T-lymphocyte cells. After the participants lowered their weight by an average of 50 pounds, the defensive power of their T-lymphocytes almost doubled.

Reported in the *International Journal of Obesity* in 1993, this study strongly suggests that obesity leads to aberrations in the immune system. Such abnormalities may well cause the same type of imbalance in the immune system that triggers RA. Of course, weight loss is one of the symptoms of RA once it begins. But many experts believe that being overweight may cause the disease in the first place.

Ample evidence exists to support this belief. Early in the 1980s, Dr. Robert Good, a prominent American immunologist, discovered that a diet high in calories can accelerate shrinkage of the thymus gland, creating tremendous imbalances in the immune system. At roughly the same time, Dr. Stuart Berger found that many overweight patients had severe imbalances in their immune systems. Numerous other studies have clearly demonstrated that a high percentage of body fat weakens immunity so that overweight people have a higher incidence of infections than people of normal weight.

American Waistlines Have Been Expanding

There seems little doubt that excess body fat is a toxic condition that harms virtually every cell, muscle, organ and system in the body, including the immune system. Medical science now considers obesity a degenerative disease comparable with hypertension or diabetes. Yet in America today, 1 person in every 3 is seriously overweight, and the soaring obesity rate has struck every race, sex and age group.

Studies show that anyone who has gained 10 to 15 pounds since age 21, or whose waistline has gained more than 2 to 3 inches, has a greatly increased risk of being hit by heart disease, stroke, hypertension, diabetes, cancer, gallstones, sleep apnea, pulmonary disease, hormonal imbalance, immunosuppression or a blood fat abnormality than a person of normal weight. As the incidence of obesity increases, 1 American in every 3 is, or will be, at risk for developing OA during his or her lifetime.

Our national obesity epidemic has spawned a colossal weight-loss industry promoting everything from diet pills to herbs and liquid diets. All are passive therapies, and as you might expect, all have a high failure rate.

For decades, dieting has been the standard approach to losing weight. But dieting doesn't work either. Thirty million Americans are constantly on some kind of diet, and all they lose is ground. That's because dieting isn't holistic. When you're just dieting, you're not really doing what it takes to succeed at losing weight. In this case, it's merely a token therapy and it doesn't do much to access our healing-regeneration system, either.

Besides, as soon as they lose weight through dieting, most people go right back to their former diet and back comes the weight. Surveys show that only 5 percent of people who lose weight through dieting are able to keep it off for 5 years.

To really get results, to restore your weight to normal and to keep it there permanently requires a total whole-person weight-loss plan that must be maintained for life.

It begins with understanding how you gain weight and with realizing that only by developing a completely new relationship with food—coupled with a regular program of both aerobic and strength-building exercise—can you restore your weight to normal and keep it there. In the process, you should get rid of much of the pain and discomfort of OA.

Reinventing the Ideal Weight

Despite the compelling need to shed surplus pounds, most Americans are becoming heavier, not lighter. One reason is that until 1996, Americans had been grossly misinformed about the level of their ideal weight. During the previous 15 years, "ideal" weight levels had been repeatedly bumped up by flawed statistics based on insurance company mortality tables. Because smokers and people with wasting diseases like cancer die younger, insurance tables showed that people lived longer when they were 10 to 15 pounds or more heavier than their true ideal weight. The old tables also allowed more permissive weights for people over 35.

All this changed when the USDA released a brand new version of the ideal weight tables early in 1996. The new ideal weights are based on a measurement called Body Mass Index or BMI. BMI is far superior to all previous ideal weight tables because it assesses the ratio between your lean muscle mass and your body weight. This ratio indicates the extent of your body fat. It's an excellent guide to the health of your body as well as to any surplus weight—and to your chances of developing OA.

The new ideal weight guidelines are published in a graph or table in the revised *Dietary Guidelines for Americans*, which you can probably find in your local library. If you are using any earlier version, I recommend discarding it immediately. Today's ideal weights are 15 percent or more below those of previous years.

174

The new guidelines disregard age and apply equally to both adult men and women. A graph shows whether your weight is in the "healthy" range, or whether you are "moderately overweight" or "severely overweight." "When your weight enters the severely overweight range, you have a growing risk of developing OA.

The new guidelines describe ranges of weights rather than pinpointing a specific ideal weight. For example, a weight between 140 to 187 is described as healthy for a man or woman 6' tall. This is adequate for the general public. But if you have a calculator handy, you can make a much more accurate assessment of how healthy your personal weight really is. If you know your height without shoes and your weight unclothed, you can calculate your personal BMI in about 2 minutes.

How to Calculate Your Personal Body Mass Index

Step 1. Multiply your weight in pounds by 705.

Step 2. Divide the result of Step 1 by your height in inches.

Step 3. Then, divide the result of Step 2 by your height in inches.

For example, for a man or woman weighing 160 pounds and standing 5'5" in height (65 inches) the calculation is:

Step 1. 160 x 705 = 112,800
Step 2. 112,800/65 = 1735.4
Step 3. 1735.4/65 = 26.7

The resulting Body Mass Index is 26.7 To find out how healthy this is, and therefore to determine your risk of developing OA, look it up in the table on page 176.

BMI Health and Weight Assessment Table

BMI Level	Health and OA Risk Assessment
19 or below	No heart disease risk, but possible risk of osteoporosis, especially in women.
20–22	Excellent health and ideal fat/muscle ratio, with no heart disease risk.
23–25	Good health, with mildly elevated level of body fat, but low risk of most diseases.
26–27	Moderately overweight; fair health with a fairly high level of body fat, which could indicate a possible future risk of OA or heart disease, diabetes and so on.
28 or over	Seriously overweight; poor health outlook with excessive body fat, too little muscle and an above-average risk for OA, heart disease, cancer, diabetes and other diseases.
32 or over	Severely overweight; clearly unhealthy with a dangerously high level of body fat, a strong possibility of muscle atrophy and a high risk of developing OA or other life-threatening degenerative disease.

So if your BMI were 26.7, as in the example above, you would have a moderate risk of developing OA at some future date. But you would be close to the borderline. Anyone with a BMI of 28 or over has an above-average risk of developing OA, as well as more life-threatening diseases, and should begin taking immediate steps to restore his or her BMI to 25 or under.

The Only Weight-Loss Plan That Really Works

I think you can sense by now that this is an entirely new approach to weight loss; in fact, it's the only one that really works. There's no dieting or counting calories. But it does require you to eat different foods than those you've probably been used to. And it does require you to exert your muscles. If you're a woman who has been unable to lose weight, even by dieting plus aerobic exercise, the following weight-loss plan may require you to exert your muscles in a different way. *That's because the secret of losing weight lies in building up strong skeletal muscles, not in trying to shed pounds by dieting.*

It works like this.

Take Charge of Your Waistline

People try to eat their way out of stress or unhappiness by binging on sweet and fatty foods. While fat and calories are piling up in the bloodstream, their glands are releasing the stress hormones cortisol and adrenalin. Working together, these hormones cause the fat that's just been eaten to migrate to the abdomen where it forms a potbelly. Meanwhile, any surplus calories are stored as body fat.

One way to tell if you're stressed is to remove the clothing around your waist and hips and measure the smallest circumference around your waist. Don't cheat by holding your breath or sucking in your abdomen. Then measure the largest circumference around your buttocks. Divide your waist size by your hip size.

For example, let's say you measure 36 inches at the slimmest part of your waist and 40 inches at the widest part of your hips. Dividing 36 by 40 equals .9. This is your waist-to-hip ratio (WHR), and it indicates the extent of fat stored in your abdomen.

177

The Safe Upper Limit for Your Waist-to-Hip Ratio

A ratio of .95 or lower is good for men. A ratio of .8 or lower is good for women. A higher ratio indicates an unhealthy level of abdominal fat. If you have a higher ratio, it indicates that stress is causing dietary fat to make its way to your middle. Central or abdominal fat, above and around the waist, has been linked to heart disease, diabetes and increased risk of some cancers. And the higher your ratio, the greater your risk for OA.

Tummy fat, or a middle-aged spread, is unlikely to occur in people who exercise. To begin with, exercise burns off surplus calories and fat. But people who exercise also have larger muscles. Muscles are biologically active. One pound of muscle consumes about 48 calories per day, even when not used. Body fat, by comparison, burns almost zero calories per day. Anyone, whether male or female, who has maintained their lean muscle mass is extremely unlikely to become overweight.

People put on weight when they stop exercising. A few months of sedentary living is all it takes for a person's muscles to become flabby and fade. Meanwhile, the body's fat stores rise. As our muscles atrophy and shrink, their mass becomes too small to burn off the body's surplus fat and calories. Our metabolism nosedives while our BMI soars.

Your Body Mass Index is a direct indicator of the ratio between your lean muscle mass and your body fat. However, your BMI isn't something you're stuck with for life. We all have direct personal control over our BMI. And if we're willing to do what it takes to succeed, every one of us can raise our metabolic rate. We can also rebalance the muscle-to-fat composition of our bodies.

PUT OSTEOARTHRITIS TO ROUT WITH THIS WHOLE-PERSON WEIGHT-LOSS PLAN

The secret of restoring your BMI to 25 or lower—and your WHR to a healthy level—is described in the 7-step program below. All 7 steps must be used together. Look up each of the Arthritis Fighters listed below and follow the instructions for carrying them out.

Step 1. Read, adopt and practice AF#5. Follow the instructions and begin to exercise aerobically 3 or more days each week for up to 45 minutes or longer.

Step 2. Read, adopt and practice AF#7. Follow the instructions and begin to work out on strength-training machines or free weights 3 or more days each week for 45 minutes or longer. Aim, if you can, to rebuild your lean muscle mass by strengthening muscles all over your body rather than focusing only on muscles in arthritic joints. When you build up muscle in your legs, arms and shoulders, you are also flattening your tummy.

Steps 1 and 2 together will have you exercising six days a week, alternating strength-building exercises one day with an aerobic workout on the following day.

Step 3. Read, adopt and practice AF#9. Discover a smorgasbord of methods for getting the fat out of your diet.

Step 4. Read, adopt and practice AF#10. Follow the instructions and introduce more foods that grow on plants into your diet.

Step 5. Read, adopt and practice AF#16 and AF#17 and visualize yourself as thin.

Step 6. Read, adopt and practice AF#18 and learn how to transform stress into nonstress.

179

Step 7. Twice a month, recalculate your BMI and WHR and record your progress in a diary. Even a small success will boost your enabling effect and your motivation. Also record how you look and feel. In just a week or two, many overweight people begin to feel better than they have in years. It's common to experience renewed energy and soaring self-esteem. Benefits like these are all it takes to turn on your healing-regeneration system and help your arthritis disappear.

To get results, practice steps 1 through 6 simultaneously and be prepared to go all the way. Don't expect to achieve much by making such token changes as switching from high-fat to low-fat cookies. To get down to your ideal weight, you must be willing to do what it takes to succeed. That means working out on strength-training equipment, exercising aerobically at a brisk pace until you perspire, cutting high-fat foods out of your diet, eating 16 or more servings of plant-based foods each day and following the fat-cutting guidelines in AF#9.

It will all become much easier if you also learn to "see" yourself as thin, as described in AF#17 and practice the stress management techniques in AF#18.

The Drug Alternative

If all this sounds too overwhelming, consider the alternative: appetite-suppressor drugs. For seven people out of ten, diet pills do work, especially dexfenfuramine (Redux), recently approved for long-term use by the FDA. However, most are powerful prescription drugs, and one rheumatologist told me he would rather be overweight than take any diet pill for an extended period of time.

The pills control food cravings by altering brain chemistry and releasing a surplus of serotonin, a soothing neurotransmitter in the brain. By manipulating brain chemistry, however, the drugs could possibly cause long-term neurological side effects such as depression, impotence or memory impairment. As it is, they may cause diarrhea, drymouth and drowsiness. And, of course, the moment you stop taking them, your weight shoots right back up again.

There's always the possibility that a new, miraculous diet pill will appear in the future. But I wouldn't count on one appearing anytime soon. Nor would I would expect a miracle from those that exist today.

In relation to drugs, did you know that over 100 different prescription drugs are capable of causing weight gain? Among the most common fat-multipliers are antidepressants, antihypertension and allergy drugs, psychiatric or mood-changing drugs and steroid-corticosteroids. Some lower the body's metabolism, while others break the nervous system's curb on appetite.

Even if new appetite-suppressor drugs do appear, their side effects could also be intolerable. There are better ways to beat OA. One of the best is to slash the fat in your diet—a strategy described in detail in Arthritis Fighter #9.

ARTHRITIS FIGHTER #9: Fewer Pounds Spell Pain-free Joints

Most people with OA in the hips, knees, ankles or feet are overweight. Being overweight abuses these joints. Climbing or descending stairs places 6 times the body's surplus weight on each of these joints. Almost every rheumatologist agrees that losing weight can help a person with OA. This is especially true when someone who is 20 percent or more overweight loses half of his or her surplus pounds.

The health risks of being overweight have been well publicized. But instead of losing weight, the average American has gained 9 to 10 pounds over the past decade. Millions of people have cut back on red meat. But instead of eating more fruits and vegetables, they have turned to other high-fat foods like pizza, hard cheese and whole-milk ice cream.

Others have replaced foods high in fat with low-fat versions of these same foods. The problem with that is foods labeled "nonfat," "low-fat" or "fat-free" often contain just as many calories as the high-fat versions. We often assume that nonfat foods are nonfattening so we turn to nonfat versions of high-fat foods in the belief they won't make us heavier.

Calories from dietary fat turn into body fat faster than calories from carbohydrates (plant foods), and dietary fat is more likely to migrate to the belly, thighs and buttocks. But surplus calories from carbohydrates can also end up as body fat if we eat enough of them. And eat more of them we do.

The Fattening of America

Calories from fat really pack on the pounds and cause or worsen OA. Recent studies by food organizations show that most Americans are aware of the dangers of overeating calories from both fat and carbohydrates. But they ignore them when shopping or eating out. Instead of ordering a baked potato that contains only 100 calories, all from carbohydrates, they order French fries, which contain an additional 200 calories from fat.

The average American today gets 34 percent of her or his calories from fat, down from 40 percent 10 years ago. Most health advisory agencies recommend eating a diet in which a *maximum* of 30 percent of calories are from fat. Yet more people are becoming heavier. One reason is that most of us fail to notice that 30 percent is the "maximum" recommended amount and that much less is better.

Many weight-loss experts believe that 20 percent of calories from fat would be healthier, while some, like the prestigious National Research Council and the Framingham Heart Study, have suggested that 15 percent of calories from fat would be more than ample.

Few of us realize it, but, on average, each American consumes the equivalent in fat of six sticks of butter each week. That might be all right for someone performing manual labor all day, but the average American's body muscles are so unused and atrophied that they are unable to burn all the surplus fat calories in the diet.

Instead, the body stores calories from fat in fat cells in the abdomen, buttocks and thighs. And since most overweight people don't exercise aerobically, calories from carbohydrates aren't burned either. So the excess is deposited as additional flab all over the body.

I've already described the pressing need to develop the body's musculature to raise the metabolism high enough to burn all the surplus calories we consume. However, this Arthritis Fighter is about cutting out the fat, and surplus carbohydrate calories, so that they don't enter our bodies in the first place.

18 NATURAL WAYS TO GET THE FAT OUT OF YOUR DIET

Step 1. To lose weight, we must recognize that eating nonfat ice cream is not the best substitute for eating regular, high-fat ice cream. It's better to replace all high-fat foods

183

with fresh fruits and vegetables. Most nonfat crackers, soups, ice cream or cheese contain nothing but empty calories. In many cases, the fat has been replaced with sugar. Few nonfat processed foods contain any of the disease-fighting fiber, antioxidants or phytomins found in fresh fruits and vegetables. (For an explanation, see AF#10.)

Step 2. You can slash from one-half to two-thirds of the fat in almost any recipe without noticing the difference. For instance, in recipes for muffins and other baked goods, substitute applesauce for 100 percent of the shortening. That works for everything except cookies.

Step 3. Be aware of the relatively high fat content of supposedly low-fat milk or other dairy products. For instance, 2-percent milk gets 35 percent of its calories from fat, while 1 percent milk still gets 23 percent of calories from fat. Instead, switch to nonfat dairy products like skim milk, powdered nonfat milk or skim milk buttermilk, or use nonfat cottage cheese or sour cream or plain nonfat yogurt. Never eat fruit-flavored yogurt or ice cream made with whole-milk products, and avoid frozen yogurt look-alikes that are often loaded with fat or sugar.

Step 4. Avoid buying convenience foods such as prepared, processed, manufactured, canned or packaged foods that line most supermarket shelves. Replace them with fresh fruits and vegetables. Half the food eaten in America is mass-produced convenience food loaded with fat and salt and ready to pop into the microwave or oven.

Step 5. Avoid foods made of refined carbohydrates like white flour, white bread or sugar and other sweeteners. Buy only bread that is clearly labeled "100 percent whole wheat" and strictly avoid most commercially produced cakes, croissants, doughnuts, muffins, pastries, pies and cookies. Most children's breakfast cereals are simply candy in disguise, and so are many similar cereals slanted at adults. Eat only breakfast cereals consisting of 100 percent whole grain with no added sugar or other sweeteners.

Step 6. Avoid the meat, deli, dairy and processed foods sections in your supermarket and focus on the produce section. If you must buy meat, tenderloin and round or flank cuts of beef are the lowest in fat. Also low are range-bred, low-fat beef, wild game and sliced turkey or chicken breast. Before cooking, cut away all visible fat and remove all poultry skin. Your total daily intake from all flesh foods except fish should never exceed 3.5 ounces of very lean meat and/ or poultry—the equivalent in size to a pack of playing cards.

Step 7. Replace meat with plant-based meat substitutes such as tempeh or plain tofu, tofu hot dogs or soy or grain-based hamburger. Soy does contain fat, but it is a far healthier version than the saturated fat found in meat. It is also believed to help prevent prostate and certain other cancers.

Step 8. Steam, bake, boil, broil, poach, stir-fry or sauté but never, never fry anything or eat any food that has been fried. Frying is a guaranteed way to turn a healthy food into a fat-laden promoter of OA and a score of other serious diseases. Vegetables like carrots, broccoli, spinach or eggplant are all virtually fat-free. But when fried, they act as sponges. A single serving can sop up 3 teaspoons of fat, equivalent to adding 135 calories—all from fat. Instead, stir-fry these and other vegetables or sauté them using a nonstick spray or a defatted broth instead of oil. *Never forget that all cooking oils are 100 percent fat!*

Step 9. Millions of Americans choose healthy, low-fat foods, but then smother them with high-fat dressings or sauces. Or they'll take a low-fat slice of wholewheat bread and plaster it with butter, margarine or mayonnaise. It's the same way with potatoes. A large baked potato, including the

185

skin, usually weighs over half a pound and has almost zero fat. But put on butter or some regular sour cream, and it swiftly adds up to 21 grams of fat, which means that 46 percent of calories are from fat. Turn the potato into chips and the original fat-free potato now has 60 percent of its calories from fat. It's difficult to believe that Americans are really sincere about losing weight when we learn that 65 percent of all potatoes in this country end up as fries, chips or hash browns, all drenched with fat. All too often it's not our food that makes us heavier but what we put on it.

Step 10. Cook low-fat and low-calorie. To enjoy authentic gourmet cooking without meat or fat, we must turn to the great culinary traditions of countries like China, India, Italy or Japan. Libraries and bookshops abound with cookbooks describing how to prepare the stir-fries of China, the curries of South India, the pastas of Italy, or the bouillabaisse of Provence. Predominantly grain-based and low in fat, the dishes of these countries offer peak experiences in taste and enjoyment with all the rich, subtle flavors and pungent seasonings that have made their cuisines famous around the world.

Step 11. Eating only foods that grow on plants can beat an addiction to fat or sugar. To do it, make your first course at each meal exclusively plant-based. For example, begin each meal with a green vegetable salad with nonfat dressing, a medium-sized bowl of vegetable soup or a bowl of whole-wheat pasta. Linger over this dish for a few minutes. By the time you're ready for the high-fat, meat-centered main course, you'll find your cravings are already satisfied and your hunger for meat and fat has largely evaporated.

Another good way to reduce your desire for fat or meat is to drink 64 ounces of liquids such as water, skim milk, black, green or herbal tea or low-calorie fruit juices each day. Sip 2 to 3 ounces at a time throughout the day.

Step 12. We're constantly exhorted to overeat, especially in restaurants. Food watchers report that serving sizes are 20 percent larger than a decade ago and most people ignore nutritional advice when they eat out, even though they're well aware of it. We still choose French fries over a baked potato. Almost everyone munches away on bread, rolls or hors d'oeuvres while waiting for the first course. All-you-can-eat meals are a real calorie buster.

The solution: Never go to a restaurant feeling hungry or eat to get your money's worth. Eat a small salad or one or two pieces of fruit at home to cut your appetite before you head for a restaurant. Otherwise, go to a restaurant with a large salad bar, order a large baked potato and use a nonfat dressing. Or try vegetables with steamed rice at a Chinese restaurant or a low-fat pasta dish with vegetables at an Italian restaurant. Remember that even in natural-food restaurants, dishes may have a high content of cheese or oil.

Step 13. How can you tell if your fat intake is 20 percent or less of your calories? A rough guide is to restrict fats and oils to only 10 percent of the weight of the total food you eat. However, that's not always easy because fats and oils lurk in dozens of processed and flesh foods.

A simpler way is to double the amount of foods from plants in your diet and halve the amount of flesh foods, dairy products and eggs. Aim to eat daily at least 5 servings of fresh vegetables, raw or cooked, 4 or more servings of fresh fruits, 6 to 11 servings of whole grains and 1 serving of legumes. This provides a total of 16 servings of unprocessed plant foods each day. From then on, the more plant-based foods and the fewer flesh foods, dairy products or eggs you eat, the sooner your Body Mass Index will reach a healthy level.

Step 14. The earlier in the day a food is eaten, the less likely it is to end up as body fat. So make breakfast the largest meal of the day. Lunch should be moderate in size, followed by a relatively light dinner. For breakfast, I eat a 100 percent whole grain cereal, often oatmeal (my cereal usually totals 2-3 servings), with 4 fresh fruits such as a banana, kiwi, apple or pear and a large slice of cantaloupe — a total of 6 or more servings of plant-based foods.

Step 15. Graze, don't gorge. Humans' early ancestors seldom ate a full meal. Instead, they "grazed," snacking on berries, tubers or fruits as they gathered them. Research shows that eating this way reduces much of the fat storage that occurs when we eat 3 main meals per day. For it to work, though, we must "graze" on plant foods just as our ancestors did, namely by eating high-fiber, low-fat fruits, vegetables, whole grains, legumes and a few nuts and seeds.

Several small studies have clearly demonstrated that when overweight people change to a mini-meal routine, they can lose an average of 2 pounds per week without cutting calories. In other words, you continue to eat the same quantity of food as you normally would in 3 main meals, but you break it into 6 or 9 smaller meals, eaten at more frequent intervals.

For a working person, it's most practical to eat hot mini-meals at home and to take snacks to eat during midmorning and midafternoon breaks and at lunchtime. Recommended snacks include plain, air-popped popcorn, rice cakes with banana, sunflower seeds and raisins, an apple or other fruit or celery or carrot sticks. Once a week, or once a day if you like, reward yourself with a fruit cocktail consisting of a mango, banana, kiwi and pear topped with plain nonfat yogurt.

Step 16. Rethink what a plate of food looks like. Anyone who has changed to a plant-based diet quickly learns that you can get the same taste enjoyment from different foods. Meat doesn't have to be the centerpiece of a dish, and fruit is often tastier than ice cream.

Most problems concerned with changing to a low-fat diet have more to do with the people we eat with than with taste. Millions of Americans still view beans and rice or vegetables as peasant food, fit only for people in Third World countries (who, incidentally, are seldom overweight). Somehow, these foods aren't socially acceptable in our affluent society. Others view a plant-based diet as restrictive and frugal, and they make up for it by going on frequent binges.

Besides, how are you going to explain to friends and family that you no longer eat the same foods they enjoy? For women, this is usually not a big problem since dieting is common. If you're male, however, you may have to announce that your doctor has ordered you to eat a low-fat diet. Most people are so in awe of doctors that this is usually all it takes.

Step 17. Watch out for high-fat sandwiches. Thousands of delis and sandwich shops across the country sell sandwiches literally loaded with fat and salt. Some sandwiches contain 5 to 8 ounces of meat, plus unknown amounts of butter. Others are loaded with processed meats. In fact, it's next to impossible to tell exactly what any sandwich contains. A tuna sandwich with mayo often contains more fat than a Big Mac. Vegetarian sandwiches may be made with wholewheat bread, but they can be filled with hard cheese.

The solution: Fill your sandwich from a salad bar, using either wholewheat bread or wholewheat pita bread.

Step 18. Don't let rumors or misinformation keep you from losing weight. Here are several important answers to common questions which prevent people from regaining a healthful BMI.

Q: Could I have inherited a fat gene?
A: One American in three is said to have inherited a gene that causes a fat-burning impairment. To many overweight

189

people, this means that fate has handed them a metabolism that burns fat too slowly to lose weight and they are doomed by their genes to be overweight for life.

In reality, very few Americans are helpless victims of an obesity gene. Regardless of your heritage, you can speed up your metabolism and lose weight if you exercise and avoid fat. Everyone who has allowed their muscles to become flabby and weak by spurning exercise has a fat-burning impairment. They have simply lost the muscle that used to burn fat.

Our real predisposition to obesity comes from inheriting a world of plenty where a myriad machines make it increasingly difficult to exert our muscles. One American in three is severely overweight because we ride everywhere by car, use a riding mower or hire a youth to mow the lawn, play golf from a cart and rarely ever walk anywhere or move fast enough to raise a sweat or our pulse.

Even if we inherited a potbelly gene, we can easily offset it. By starting a regular program of both aerobic and strength-building exercise, and by getting the fat out of our diet, chances are good that any fat-burning impairment will start to disappear in just a short time. But until we begin this program, we'll continue to hoard fat.

If you still believe you have inherited a fat-burning impairment, have your doctor monitor you at the same time as you read, adopt and practice AF#5, 7, 8 and 10.

Q: Is it dangerous to cut back on dietary fat if you are insulin-resistant?

A: During periods of abundance, humans always stored surplus calories in the body's fat layers as insurance against future food shortages. Although primitive humans scavenged or hunted flesh foods, its fat content was low and most of their diet consisted of foods that grow on plants. Most plant foods are composed of carbohydrates, and that includes not only pasta, potatoes, rice and fat-free desserts, but also lettuce and just about all fruits, vegetables, legumes, grains, seeds and nuts. To transform a carbohydrate into energy, and to store it in the muscles and in the body's fat layers, the pancreas must secrete the hormone insulin.

The insulin-resistance theory is that during periods of food abundance—as in modern America—the pancreas overproduces insulin to convert carbohydrate into energy and fat. According to this theory, much of the carbohydrates we eat end up adding to our fat reserves. Since modern humans are rarely, if ever, faced with a food shortage, these fat stores are never depleted. They simply remain as unsightly flab on the abdomen, buttocks and thighs.

If we cut back on fat and eat more carbohydrates in an effort to lose weight, so much extra insulin is required that the pancreas is swiftly overloaded. According to this theory, when someone tries to replace too many fat calories with carbohydrate calories, the pancreas may experience burnout. This translates into an increased risk of diabetes or heart disease.

For millions of Americans this theory has merely reinforced the belief that being overweight is beyond their control. After all, how can you lower the fat content of your diet if doing so puts you at risk for a dangerous disease?

Most weight-loss experts consider this theory extremely controversial and a wonderful excuse for millions of Americans to continue eating a high-fat diet.

To begin with, the theory totally ignores the need for exercise. Almost all cases of insulin resistance exist in overweight people with flabby, atrophied muscles who haven't exercised in years. When people who are insulin-resistant rebuild their muscles with exercise, their new, larger muscles can store far more energy from carbohydrate foods. These larger muscles also boost their metabolism by burning calories 24 hours a day. When hundreds of additional calories are burned each day by aerobic exercise, the body's need for insulin is dramatically reduced. And insulin resistance no longer exists.

As this was written, the consensus of informed opinion was that eating a high proportion of foods from carbohydrates does not make a person who is insulin-resistant overweight. To become overweight, you must eat more calories than the body burns as energy.

The solution to insulin resistance is not to cut back on plant-based foods and keep on eating fat. The answer is to restore your lean muscle mass with a combination of strength-training and aerobic exercise.

Simultaneously, we need to stop eating white bread, white flour and sugar. Instead, we need to reduce our intake of fat and eat more high-fiber plant foods like barley, beans, carrots, potatoes, prunes, yams, apples and citrus that dampen the insulin response. High-fiber foods like these fill you up without overloading the body with calories.

Most Americans eat a diet pitifully deficient in fiber. And most overweight people consume fewer than 11 grams of fiber daily versus the recommended 25 to 35 grams. Moreover, digesting carbohydrates consumes 25 calories per 100 calories of plant-based foods, while it takes only 3 calories of energy to digest 100 calories of fat. Obviously, the more foods you eat that grow on plants, the more you drive up your metabolism.

If you believe you are insulin-resistant, have your doctor confirm it. Then turn back to AF#8 and read, adopt and practice the Whole-Person Weight-Loss Plan while your doctor monitors your progress. As your weight begins to drop, your insulin resistance should also begin to fade.

Meanwhile, don't fall into the trap of believing you are

destined to always be overweight because you are insulin-resistant. There is a way out that works. All that's required is to use your mind and muscles to do what it takes to succeed.

Q: Why do I eat when I'm not really hungry?
A: The most likely reason is that you're using food as a tranquilizer. We often eat because we're bored, worried, unhappy, pressured or feeling anxious, lonely or unloved. When we eat a candy bar or drink a sugar-filled soda, it triggers an immediate rise in our blood sugar level that creates a temporary relief from our problems.

When we eat for psychological reasons, we respond to cues such as the crunchiness or the aroma or the texture or the sizzle of food. These cues bring up childhood memories of when Mom gave us sweet or fatty foods to make us feel content and happy. When we're adults, we crave these same pleasant feelings and memories. We do so by craving the same sweet and fatty foods that help us to retrieve these memories. And we overeat them to the point of substance abuse. Soon we are as hooked on these foods as an alcoholic is on liquor or a smoker on cigarettes.

The solution: When a craving arises, stop. Take 10 slow, deep breaths. Realize that you aren't actually hungry. You don't need the potato chips, the ice cream or the steak. You simply crave the crunchiness or the creamy texture or the sizzle and the memories they bring back. Then immediately do something that is incompatible with eating, like taking a quick walk around the block. The realization that much of our overeating is purely psychological, and not because we're hungry, is enough for most people to break this form of substance abuse.

Q: What can I do? Once I start eating certain foods, I can't stop until I've eaten all there is.
A: As in the preceding answer, we may develop an addiction

to certain binge foods. Almost always these are high-fat, high-calorie foods we've eaten since Mom gave them to us as youngsters to keep us pacified. Down through the years, certain events have triggered a craving for these foods. While watching TV or a ball game, we often binge on cheese snacks or potato chips, completely unaware of the amount we are eating.

We can put a stop to binging like this in four easy steps.

1. Make a list of all the foods you binge on. Typically, they might include ice cream; candies or chocolate; cookies, cakes or doughnuts; potato chips or crackers; cheese or cheese snacks; pizza or fried chicken.

2. Recognize that you binge on these problem foods in response to a trigger situation or event. So make a list of the situations that cause you to reach for a binge food and eat it all. Typical trigger situations are watching TV, writing creatively or working on a report, socializing at a party, eating in a restaurant or talking on the telephone.

3. Stop buying binge foods and keep them out of your house. Replace them with healthier, low-fat snack foods like plain air-popped popcorn or fruit. If you must buy a binge food, purchase only the smallest amount so that you cannot keep on eating.

4. Avoid eating during or immediately after a trigger situation. For example, never eat standing up or while on the phone. At parties, avoid finger foods except fruits, vegetables or other healthy, low-fat snacks. Then pick them up only with your nondominant hand. It's also a good idea not to send out for food, if you can avoid it.

Above all, never let a binge food control you to the point where you can't control the amount you eat.

Losing weight won't cure osteoarthritis. But if you have

194

OA in a weight-bearing joint, getting back to your ideal weight may relieve much of the stress and pain. The next Arthritis Fighter completes the strategy for beating OA through nutrition. It could also be a vital therapy for anyone with gout or RA.

ARTHRITIS FIGHTER #10: The One Diet That Does It All

The one diet that does it all can help beat arthritis in three different ways:

- It can help normalize weight in people whose OA or gout is caused by being overweight.
- It can simplify the diet of people with gout and replace purine-rich foods with healthier fare.
- It may help alleviate the pain and symptoms of RA in people who have a mild-to-moderate level of the disease.

It can also cut your risk of dying from heart disease or cancer by up to 90 percent, and it can help prevent almost every other disease or dysfunction.

Yet this incredible nutritional breakthrough is not really a diet at all. It's simply a different way of eating that focuses on foods that help your body and avoids foods that harm it.

In other words, it's a plant-based diet, meaning it's composed exclusively of foods that grow on plants such as fruits, vegetables, whole grains, legumes, nuts and seeds. The term "plant-based" is used nowadays in preference to "vegetarian," since so many so-called vegetarians eat high-fat dairy foods, eggs and often fish or poultry as well.

The Arthritis-Fighting Power of Plant-based Foods

For decades, it's been observed that a changeover to a plant-based diet has effectively ended many cases of RA. Despite the strong links discovered between diet and heart disease or cancer, most rheumatologists have continued to deny any link between diet and RA. That is, until patients with heart disease, who also had RA, were ordered to make dietary changes to lower their risk of a heart attack. The changes consisted of eating many more fruits and vegetables each day, while slashing their intake of foods high in fat such as flesh foods, whole-milk dairy products and eggs.

In numerous cases, these heart disease patients reported not only less chest pain from angina but a significant reduction in the pain and symptoms of RA. Other studies have confirmed that the more plant-based foods we eat, and the fewer foods of animal origin, the greater the improvement in RA symptoms.

For example, a Norwegian study published in the *British Journal of Nutrition* (November 1994) revealed that a plant-based diet eased the pain and symptoms of RA in most of the 23 participants who formed the test group. Prior to the study, each of these participants had eaten a conventional meat-based diet all their lives.

The test group then followed an exclusively plant-based diet with no flesh foods, dairy products, eggs or wheat for 3.5 months. They then added small amounts of eggs and dairy products back into their diet and continued to eat this way for the next 9 months.

Throughout the 12.5-month duration of the study, a control group of 21 people matched for age, sex and RA symptoms continued to eat a conventional meat-based diet. None showed any improvement. But the 23 people in the test group experienced a significant reduction in RA pain, morning stiffness, joint tenderness and swelling. Five were able to reduce intake of NSAIDs while on the plant-based diet.

During a follow-up survey one year later, researchers found that 16 of the original 23 had adopted a plant-based diet permanently. These 16 continued to report reduced pain and symptoms. The explanation: Study authors suspect that benefits were due to a higher intake of antioxidants and a reduced intake of rogue molecules called free radicals that abound in fat and meat.

Plants Against Arthritis

A plant-based dict doesn't help everyone with RA, but in similar studies in Finland, Sweden and the Netherlands, most participants reported that their RA pain and symptoms improved

In the Swedish study, authored by Lars Skoldstam at Sundvalls Hospital in Sundvalls, a group of 20 men and women with RA stayed on a plant-based diet for 4 months, after which 11 reported feeling considerably better. The author concluded that a plant-based diet may help about half of all people with mild-to-moderate RA feel better—which is about as much as most drugs do.

The Finnish study examined the possible power of antioxidants to prevent RA. Blood samples were taken from 1,420 participants showing their levels of the antioxidant vitamins C and E and the mineral selenium. Over a 20-year period, those with the lowest antioxidant levels were 8 times more likely to develop RA than those with the highest levels (reported in *Annals of Rheumatic Diseases*, vol. 53, 1994).

A diet high in fruits and vegetables and low in foods of animal origin has been confirmed as the single best way to prevent heart disease, stroke, cancer, diabetes, kidney disease and obesity. Each of these is a degenerative disease and the majority of Americans die of one of these diseases.

RA, OA and gout are among nonfatal degenerative diseases. More and more health professionals are beginning to suspect that a plant-based diet may also be the best defense against most forms of arthritis.

Because it is low in fat and high in fiber, a plant-based diet benefits overweight people with gout or OA by helping them normalize their weight. Foods that grow on plants also contain nutrients that may help prevent further damage to cartilage in joints.

How Free Radicals Create Chemical Havoc in the Body

Whenever we eat high-fat foods of animal origin, we release huge numbers of unstable and reactive molecules called "free radicals." These renegade molecules roam the body, damaging vital cell structures and enzymes. In the process, some researchers suspect that free radicals are also responsible for the chemical havoc that destroys cartilage, bone and muscle in arthritic joints.

Free radicals are released from saturated fat found primarily in foods of animal origin and from polyunsaturated vegetable oils such as corn, safflower, soybean, cottonseed and sunflower oil. Another rich source of free radicals is partially hydrogenated vegetable oil, a manufactured oil found in margarine and almost every form of commercial baked goods and processed foods. Cigarette smoking remains the most potent producer of free radicals in existence, which is one reason why smokers have a far higher incidence of RA than nonsmokers.

It is these free radicals from high-fat foods and cigarettes that are responsible for millions of deaths every year from heart disease and cancer.

Antioxidants in Plant Foods Snuff Out Free Radicals

Eating at least 9 servings of fruits and vegetables each day, plus several servings of whole unrefined grains and at least one serving of legumes, is nature's answer to the free-radical threat. That's because the function of plants is to oxidize carbon into carbohydrate using solar energy. In the process, plants release huge amounts of free radicals into their tissues. Yet plants are virtually immune to free-radical damage. The reason is that plants produce enormous quantities of natural antioxidants that sop up and neutralize free radicals.

By eating an abundance of foods that grow on plants, we absorb such generous amounts of these same antioxidants that free-radical damage is slowed to a crawl inside our bodies.

But there are other huge pluses to eating plant foods. Almost all plant foods are low in fat and high in fiber, a nutrient that prevents obesity and a long list of other diseases. Plant foods are equally rich in other disease-fighting substances called "phytomins" or "phytochemicals." While phytomins help protect the body from many life-threatening diseases, it is too early to definitely say whether they offer any protection from arthritis.

However, the need for fruits and vegetables in the diet goes way beyond our requirements for vitamins or minerals. Only now are researchers coming to realize the tremendous power of phytomins in preventing and retarding the progress of modern humanity's most dangerous diseases.

Whether or not you have arthritis, everyone needs to eat many more fruits and vegetables each day and far fewer foods of animal origin. So many hundreds of disease-fighting phytomins exist in plant foods that researchers have yet to identify them all. So far, 14 categories of phytomins have been classified, including carotenoids, flavonoids, indoles, phenols, phylates and sulfides. Many of these are also antioxidants.

Buttress Your Diet with Phytomins

Among the best sources of both phytomins and antioxidants are apricots, bananas, bok choy, broccoli, Brussels sprouts, cabbage, carrots, cauliflower, celery, citrus, cucumbers, dried beans-peas-lentils, eggplant, garlic, greens of all types, kale, kiwi fruit, mangoes, melons—especially cantaloupes and watermelon—nuts, onions, parsley, parsnips, peppers, persimmons, pineapples, potatoes, pumpkin, rutabagas, seeds—especially sunflower seeds—soybeans and tofu (a curd made from soybeans), spinach, squash, strawberries, sweet potatoes, tomatoes, turnips and whole grains, especially oats and wheat germ.

By comparison, no food of animal origin contains any fiber, antioxidants or phytomins and relatively few vitamins or minerals. Except for calcium in dairy products, most meat, chicken, fish and eggs constitute a nutritional wasteland. The fat and protein they do contain is probably the last thing the average American needs. The same could be said of sugar, white flour, white bread and most other plant foods that have been depleted of their nutrients through manufacturing, processing or refining.

The closer plant foods are to their original, natural state, the richer they are in nutrients that may help to prevent or retard degenerative diseases, including arthritis. Cooking doesn't destroy the fiber in beans or grains. But it can deplete the nutrients in vegetables. Steaming, baking or microwaving causes the least nutritional damage. But whenever possible, vegetables are best eaten raw in a salad.

With few exceptions, it's difficult to eat too many plant foods. One exception: If you're trying to lose weight, go easy on avocadoes, beans, nuts and seeds. Otherwise, these are among the most healthful of foods.

A Brave New Eating Plan That May Benefit Arthritis

Space limitations prevent describing in detail exactly how to maximize plant foods in your diet. Personally, for breakfast I eat a whole grain cereal such as oatmeal or shredded wheat with 4 fresh fruits; lunch is a green salad, composed of lettuce, avocado, shredded carrots, cucumber, green onions, tomato, sprouted or boiled soybeans, bell peppers or celery with a dressing of plain nonfat yogurt or perhaps tofu; and dinner features steamed or baked vegetables such as potatoes, sweet potatoes, onions, broccoli or greens, or maybe a grain-based dish with vegetables, while dessert is a cocktail of fresh fruit with a topping of plain nonfat yogurt.

If we're away from home at lunch, we take homemade sandwiches with sunflower seeds and raisins, and we try to avoid eating in restaurants unless they have a salad bar. (For more tips on healthful eating see AF#9.)

A word of advice: To avoid bloating or flatulence, ease your way into a plant-based diet. At first, make every second meal plant-based while you continue to eat conventional but less fatty meals in between. As your digestive system becomes more accustomed to high-fiber foods, all of your meals can consist of foods that grow on plants.

To minimize gas, soak all legumes before cooking. Discard the soaking water. And avoid mixing beans with cabbage family vegetables. Remember, too, that high-fiber foods often require more chewing than other foods. Since fiber sponges up water from the intestines, drink at least 6 to 8 glasses of fluid daily.

Most healthy people can make the transition to eating 30 grams of fiber daily in 3 or 4 weeks. But if you have a bowel disorder or kidney disease, if you could possibly develop a blocked bowel or have had recent surgery or if you have any other type of gastrointestinal tract disorder, you need medical clearance before changing your diet.

Fight Back with a Better Diet

Altogether, I've seen at least 20 different "Arthritis Diets." They can't all work. The only one for which I've seen any valid proof is a diet composed exclusively of foods that grow on plants. The plant-based diet has been endorsed by a score of health advisory services, including the National Research Council, the Framingham Heart Study and the American Diabetic Association.

Adding fruits and vegetables to any diet can only make it healthier. Incorporate a plant-based diet into a whole-person approach, together with exercise and stress management, and even if it doesn't improve your arthritis, it will help normalize your weight, prevent most diseases, retard the aging process and improve your health—truly the one diet that does it all.

ARTHRITIS FIGHTER #11: Relieve Rheumatoid Arthritis with a Natural Food from the Sea

---

New studies are showing that the inflammation and morning stiffness caused by RA can be increased by eating meat and other high-fat foods of animal origin and decreased by eating fatty fish or certain foods that grow on plants. It all depends on the type of fat we're eating.

Fat is composed of building blocks called "fatty acids." These same fatty acids are also the building blocks (precursors) of prostaglandins. In turn, prostaglandins are hormone-like substances that can promote or control inflammation and a host of other body functions. For example, the prostaglandin Leukotriene B4 is a powerful promoter of inflammation. Leukotriene B4 production is intensified by eating arachidonic acid, a fatty acid found principally in meat and other foods of animal origin.

But other prostaglandins are powerful anti-inflammatory agents. By inhibiting production of Leukotriene B4, these "good" prostaglandins help relieve inflammation and stiffness in thousands of people with RA.

The precursors of these "good" prostaglandins are two Omega-3 fatty acids. EPA (or eicosapentaenoic acid) is found primarily in fatty fish, while GLA (or gamma linolenic acid) is found primarily in evening primrose oil.

These discoveries came about when researchers analyzed a series of small but careful studies that linked consumption of various fats with the pain and symptoms experienced by people with RA. The studies emanated from as far afield as Scotland and Australia. But the most consistent work was done by Joel M. Kremer, M.D., head of the Division of Rheumatology at Albany Medical College, N.Y., and the leading researcher on the link between fish oil and RA.

The consensus of these studies is that when people with class 1 or 2 (mild-to-moderate) RA replace the meat in their diet with fatty fish, approximately one-third experience a significant reduction in inflammation, morning stiffness and fatigue. However, researchers caution against expecting a miracle. You have to eat the oily fish 5 days a week for several weeks or months before appreciable benefits appear. And eating fatty fish seldom cures RA completely.

Pain Relief Without Drugs

Nonetheless, this is exciting news for anyone bothered by the headaches, stomach upset and other adverse side effects caused by NSAIDs. Several studies showed that eating fatty fish reduced pain and inflammation in at least 1 person in 3 by approximately the same extent as taking pain-killing NSAID drugs. For example, the most recent study from Albany Medical College, reported in *Arthritis and Rheumatism* (August 1995), concluded that people with RA tolerated coming off NSAIDs better after having taken fish oil supplements for approximately 5 months.

When the results of all the studies were pooled, another important finding was that, with the exception of EPA and GLA fatty acids and of olive, canola and flaxseed oils, almost all other fats and oils are likely to worsen RA.

Yet another finding is that a high-fat diet aggravates painful swelling and stiffness in people with RA, while a diet low in fat may dramatically reduce these symptoms. One very small study at Wayne State University found that after 7 weeks on a low-fat diet, inflammation and swelling had decreased by 75 percent. When participants returned to a high-fat diet, their RA symptoms returned within 72 hours.

Nathan Pritikin and other heart disease researchers found that a very low-fat diet reduced RA symptoms in 90 percent of people with RA in the hands, fingers or wrists and 50 percent in people with RA in the knees and hips.

Eating Fish Beats Taking Fish-Oil Supplements

To provide better control, fish-oil supplements were used in the various studies. But virtually every author recommends eating fish rather than taking supplements. Most study authors recommend eating a serving of up to 8 ounces of oily fish 5 times a week in place of meat and all other foods of animal origin except plain, nonfat dairy foods.

Even if you do not yet have RA, eating fish once or twice a week may help prevent it. Observers at the University of

Washington in Seattle found that women who ate baked or broiled fish 1 to 2 times a week were 25 percent less likely to develop RA than women who ate fish once a week or less often. And women who ate fish 2 or more times a week were 43 percent less likely to develop RA.

The highest content of EPA fatty acids is found in fatty cold-water fish such as anchovies, bluefish, halibut, herring, Atlantic mackerel, sardines packed in water and tuna. To a lesser extent, EPA occurs in purslane, a common garden weed, in several types of beans—especially soybeans and tofu—and also in chestnuts and walnuts. (Caution: Some of these may also be high in purines and unsuitable for anyone with gout.)

The highest content of GLA is found in evening primrose oil and also in blackcurrant oil. Most studies have used oily fish since they are a familiar food and more readily obtainable than the rather exotic oils. However, GLA is also available in supplements.

Watch Out for Gremlin Fats

The same studies on fat and RA revealed other helpful facts. First, the following sources of dietary fat are likely to worsen RA: meat, especially beef, pork and lamb; all dairy products except plain nonfat; polyunsaturated vegetable oils such as corn, safflower, sesame and sunflower seed and soybean; and partially hydrogenated vegetable oils which abound in margarine, shortening and almost all commercial baked goods and processed foods. Egg yolks, fried foods, regular mayonnaise, fish roe, gravy, chocolate, candy and just about any other foods containing the "bad" fats just described are likely to worsen the symptoms of RA.

Second, while we overdose on these gremlin fats, over 60

205

percent of Americans are starved for two key essential fatty acids (EFAs), namely, linolenic and linoleic fatty acids. These EFAs play a vital role in regulating both the inflammation response and the immune response, two factors intimately linked with RA. These priceless EFAs are found in abundance in soybeans and soybean products, sunflower and sesame seeds, nuts—especially almonds, filberts and walnuts—green leafy vegetables, fish and canola, flaxseed and olive oils.

Certainly, EFAs also exist in pure polyunsaturated vegetable oils such as soybean, sunflower or safflower oils. But the refined oils sold in supermarkets have often been so heated, bleached, degummed and deodorized that the biochemical content of their EFAs may be altered. For this reason, flaxseed oil is considered the purest source of EFAs.

Most nutritionists suggest that 1 tablespoon of flaxseed oil per day is sufficient for a healthy person, but anyone with RA may need two. Taking 1 tablespoon per day would seem prudent if you are on an exclusively plant-based diet. If you smoke, however, you should know that smoking completely destroys any linoleic acid in the bloodstream.

Can Eating Fish Help People with Osteoarthritis?

How do all these findings about fat affect anyone with OA or gout? Certainly, everyone needs an adequate intake of EFAs each day. Otherwise, if you're overweight, all the "bad" fats should be avoided and—if they're making you overweight—some of the "good" fats as well.

Fish is the least harmful of flesh foods; therefore it's a good substitute for meat, eggs or poultry. Yet if you don't have RA, low-fat fish may be as beneficial as fish that are high in oil and fat. Or you may be better off without any flesh foods at all (see AF#10).

In conclusion, cut back on certain foods or fats, and maintain your weight at, or slightly above, your ideal weight by increasing your intake of more desirable foods such as fruits, vegetables, beans, whole grains and nonfat dairy products. Don't take prophylactic aspirin to prevent heart disease with a diet of oily fish. And try to avoid taking cod liver oil—it's dangerously high in vitamins A and D.

ARTHRITIS FIGHTER #12: When Troublemaking Foods May Cause "Arthritis"

"It was my diary that led me to the cause of my rheumatoid arthritis," said Jennifer, a 35-year-old Chicago bank teller. "Every morning when I woke up with my fingers so stiff and bent I could not hold a pen, my diary told me that the day before I'd always eaten tomatoes or potatoes or peppers or some other food of the nightshade family. Since then, I've avoided nightshade foods and I've had no more rheumatoid arthritis. I'm sure it was the acid in these foods that caused the problem."

Sound familiar?

While researching this book, I met at least a dozen people who had recovered from RA by eliminating one or more foods from their diet, and I heard or read of hundreds more. The problem with their stories is that not one of them had ever been medically diagnosed with RA. Only 5 had been medically examined, and none of these had any trace of rheumatoid factor, a substance which usually confirms the existence of RA.

Nor was there any clear agreement as to which foods might be the cause of RA flare-ups. Moreover, before eliminating the foods that relieved their RA, each of the people with whom I spoke had previously read or heard that RA was triggered by eating certain foods, especially wheat, corn, beef, dairy products, eggs, sugar and nightshade family foods.

For years, books and magazine articles have been telling readers that RA may be triggered by eating certain foods. By now, almost everyone who has RA is aware that the disease may be due to a food allergy. In other words, they could already have built up a strong faith and belief that their RA would improve if they cut out one or more of the gremlin foods from their diet.

Could a Special Diet Help Your RA?

In 1986, Dr. Richard Panush, chief of the division of chemical immunology at the University of Florida College of Medicine in Gainesville, tested a group of people with RA and found that only 3 percent experienced any pain relief when placed on foods reputed to benefit RA.

But during a followup study, 30 percent of the participants still thought that their RA was aggravated by certain foods. Dr. Panush then gave each of them that food without their knowledge. Only a very small number reported any increase in pain or symptoms of RA.

While the study failed to show any link between food allergy and RA, it did demonstrate that when patients tend to view food as the cause of RA they are likely to avoid exercise and other therapies that might really help. For example, unless you have a bona-fide allergy to lactose in milk, cutting out dairy products could deprive you of needed calcium.

Molecular biologists have given us a new understanding of food allergies so that nowadays food as a cause of RA is considered controversial and mostly just theory. Extensive tests have shown that, at most, fewer than 4 percent of people with medically diagnosed RA are biochemically sensitive to certain foods. When RA symptoms have improved after a dietary change, it has almost always been due to switching to a low-fat or plant-based diet, eating oily fish, increasing essential fatty acids, being taken off medication, the placebo effect or not having genuine RA in the first place.

A Food Intolerance That Mimics Arthritis

Some studies have continued to show that certain foods provoke what appears to be an RA flare-up in some people. On closer analysis, it was found that these people rarely had medically diagnosed RA. Instead, they had a condition known as "allergic arthritis" which mimics some of the symptoms of RA. When the offending food or foods are eliminated, allergic arthritis disappears.

Allergic arthritis is actually an allergy triggered by the aberrant functioning of the immune system. An out-of-balance immune system may react to harmless dust, ragweed, cat hairs, pollen or food molecules with a variety of symptoms, ranging from asthma to hives, mood swings or depression, a runny nose or inflammation.

The link between food and allergic arthritis affects people either who have an unusually thin mucosal lining in their digestive tract or whose mucosal lining has been irritated and inflamed by repeated doses of certain NSAID painkilling drugs.

When such a person consumes a large amount of one type of food, say, potatoes, incompletely digested potato molecules are absorbed through the mucosal lining into the bloodstream. Immediately, receptors on these food cells are recognized by the immune system as foreign. The body's immune response is triggered and IgG antibodies attach

209

themselves to the potato cells to form a circulating immune complex. This complex is then carried by the bloodstream throughout the body.

Food Foes May Cause Inflammation

If the complex lodges in a blood vessel wall, it causes vasculitis or hives. If it lodges in the synovium, or inner lining of a joint, it creates inflammation and other symptoms that mimic those of RA. Eventually, the complex is removed by large macrophage scavenger cells. That is, until we eat another overdose of potatoes—or whatever food is triggering allergic arthritis.

When the immune system recognizes potato, or other food molecules, as threatening, it turns on part of the fight-or-flight response. The adrenals then begin to secrete stress hormones. As we keep on eating generous servings of potatoes at each meal, the adrenals become exhausted. Our blood sugar level drops and we experience fatigue.

We can develop an addiction to potatoes (or any one of a dozen other foods) just as surely as we can become addicted to cigarettes or alcohol. Unless we continue to eat the foods to which we are addicted, we soon feel listless and unable to concentrate. These, of course, are withdrawal symptoms. But we seldom experience withdrawal symptoms because we always give ourselves another fix of addictive food before that happens.

Allergic arthritis is not considered a true form of arthritis because it rarely damages a joint. Primarily, it causes inflammation and stiffness which resemble symptoms of bona-fide RA. But a food allergy rarely, if ever, causes true RA, nor, as far as anyone knows, any other type of arthritis. Nonetheless, allergic arthritis can be easily stopped by, first, identifying the food, foods or beverage causing the allergy and, second, permanently removing them from the diet.

How to Identify Foods Which May Be Causing Allergic Arthritis

To identify a food, foods or beverage to which you may be addicted, and which is responsible for allergic arthritis, answer the following questions by naming the specific foods or beverages.

1. Must you have a certain food for breakfast each morning before you feel ready to face the day?
2. Must you have a certain food at lunch or for between-meal snacks?
3. Must you eat a certain food, such as eggs, cheese or bread, in some form at every meal to feel satisfied?
4. Must you eat a certain food just before bedtime in order to fall asleep?
5. If they were no longer available, which foods would you miss most?
6. Do you always stock up on certain foods because you may feel listless or fatigued if you run out?
7. Do you experience discomfort if you are late for a meal, or if you miss a meal containing certain foods?
8. Could you relieve this discomfort by eating certain foods?
9. Does eating a certain food give you a lift, but when you can't get it, you feel listless and weak?
10. Do certain foods often cause indigestion, heartburn, gas or other digestive problems?

Typically, the foods you listed might include wheat, yeast, whole-milk dairy products, beef, pork, shrimp, smoked and processed meats, eggs and tuna. Now list them again starting with the food you crave most, eat most frequently and consume most of. Then list the remainder in decreasing order.

211

This is your list of suspected food allergens. Chances are good that one or more of the first five foods on your list is the cause of your allergic arthritis.

Don't omit alcohol from your list of suspect foods and beverages if you believe you are addicted to it. Millions of people try to ameliorate arthritis pain by having a few drinks each evening. Alcohol can easily intensify arthritis symptoms.

Test Your Food Sensitivities with an Elimination Diet

The elimination diet is probably as effective as any expensive allergy test. Some older books suggest preceding it with a fast. But nowadays fasting has fallen into disrepute. Instead, I suggest following the five steps below.

Step 1. Eliminate from your diet the first five foods and beverages on your list of suspected food allergens. Replace them with an equal amount of the following foods which are rarely allergenic: bananas, beets, broccoli, Brussels sprouts, buckwheat, cantaloupe, carrots, cauliflower, green beans, kiwi fruit, mangoes, peas, rice, sweet potatoes, tofu or turnips. Your weight should never drop below your ideal level.

Continue to eat this diet for five full days. Expect some withdrawal symptoms during this time. When you stop eating a food to which you are addicted, it's like experiencing a drug withdrawal. You may feel minor flu-like symptoms or a headache or fatigue for 1 to 3 days. If you experience what appear to be withdrawal symptoms, this supports the likelihood that one or another of the foods on your suspect list is the cause of your allergic arthritis.

Step 2. On the sixth day, eat a medium-sized serving of the first food on your list at all three meals. In all probability, you will have a swift reaction. If so, stop eating the suspect food. If not, repeat Step 2 on the seventh day.

Step 3. As soon as you get a clear and unmistakable return of allergic arthritis symptoms, note the details in a diary. Name the trigger food that appeared to set off the reaction and the symptoms you experienced, noting the date and time of each event.

Step 4. After dinner on day 7 cease testing. If the suspect food you already tested did not provoke a response, add it back into your elimination diet. If it did, eliminate it completely from your diet. Continue to eat the elimination diet on days 8 through 12.

Step 5. On day 13, repeat Step 2, testing the second food on your list. After that, continue to test one suspect food each week until you have tested all five.

If one of the first five foods on your list fails to provoke allergic arthritis, it's unlikely that any others will. In this case, your allergic arthritis may be triggered by another type of allergen.

Test One Suspect Food Each Week

Testing each of the first five foods on your list should take two months. Now go ahead and retest each of these foods once more, using exactly the same test you did the first time. A second reaction should verify that the food, or foods, may very well be the cause of your allergic arthritis.

The final step is to permanently eliminate from your diet any of the foods you have verified as allergens. Replace these foods with a variety of the rarely allergenic foods listed in *Step 1* of the elimination test. Continue to eat this allergy-free diet.

213

Retest a food several times if you have any doubts. It isn't always clear whether the pain and stiffness in your fingers on Wednesday were caused by the beef and potatoes you ate for dinner on Tuesday. In a case like this, you may have to repeat the test several times to ensure that results are consistent. Test only one food per week and eliminate it from your diet for five full days before retesting.

Do Nightshade Family Foods Really Cause Arthritis?

Several decades ago, a horticulturist at Rutgers University thought that a diet high in nightshade foods might be the cause of knee pain in cattle. Over the years, this isolated event grew into a widespread belief that nightshade family foods were responsible for RA.

Nowadays, some 30 percent of people with genuine RA experience some degree of improvement after they eliminate nightshade foods from their diets. Several prominent researchers have pointed out that 30 percent is exactly the percentage of benefit to be expected from the placebo effect. So, most of the benefit associated with cutting out nightshade foods appears to be purely psychological.

However, nightshade foods could be allergenic for someone with allergic arthritis. Since all nightshade foods are botanically related, if you have allergic arthritis and you react to any one nightshade food, it usually pays to test the others.

Nightshade family foods include eggplant, paprika, peppers—red, green or chili but not black—potatoes and tomatoes. Some people believe that all nightshade foods contain a toxin called "solanin" that provokes joint pain. If this is true, the joint pain is more likely due to allergic arthritis rather than bona-fide RA.

Various types of nightshade foods, such as potato starch or tomato paste, are widely used in processed and packaged foods. Thus it is difficult to eliminate them entirely.

Only Primary Foods Should Be Tested

For the same reason you should test only primary rather than complex foods. For example, if a hamburger provokes allergic arthritis, is it the wheat in the bun, the meat or the lettuce, tomato or onion?

If a whole hamburger triggers allergic arthritis, by all means eliminate hamburgers from your diet. Later, however, you could test each of the ingredients in the hamburger separately. Why cut out the wheat if it's the meat that is causing the problem?

A final caveat: Whenever you experiment with your diet, continue to take your medications unless you have your doctor's approval. If you have any severe allergic reactions such as asthma, epilepsy, emotional disturbances or mood swings, or if you have required medical treatment for allergies in the past, or if you have diabetes or are under a doctor's care for any condition which might be worsened by elimination and reintroduction of a food, you should have your doctor's approval before using any of the action-steps in AF#12.

ARTHRITIS FIGHTER #13: Conquer Gout Without Drugs

If you read the section "Understanding Gout" at the end of Chapter 3, you will already understand the causes of gout and how it develops. You will also have learned that, if you're willing to do what it takes to succeed, gout is one form of arthritis that most people can get rid of.

Yet 2 million Americans continue to have gout. The reason is that gout can be controlled by an oral medication. By comparison, to stop gout naturally requires a whole-person approach that calls for exercise, weight loss, a change of diet and the elimination of alcohol. Most gout sufferers prefer to take the easy way and pop a pill.

The problem with controlling gout by medication is that the sufferer remains at risk for heart disease, stroke, diabetes, cancer or OA. The person is still usually overweight, physically unattractive and in poor health to the point where his or her quality of life is impaired to some degree. The drugs may also cause drowsiness and upset stomach.

There must be a better way. And if you're willing to do what it takes to succeed, there is.

The Whole-Person, All-Natural Way to Permanently End the Pain and Symptoms of Gout Without Drugs

Just follow the following seven steps:

Step 1. Peel off the pounds and normalize your weight. Almost everyone who has gout is overweight, and a number of gout experts believe that restoring weight to normal does more to eliminate gout than anything else. Since some people with gout have borderline diabetes, any overweight gout sufferer needs to lose weight gradually. So crash dieting or fasting is strictly out. Even a very low-calorie diet could create a dramatic boost in uric acid level, causing gout symptoms to suddenly flare up.

Instead, you should lose weight slowly and gradually by cutting back on animal fats and protein over a period of weeks or months while increasing your intake of plant-based foods. The best way to do this is to read, adopt and practice AF#8: Defeat Osteoarthritis by Peeling Off the Pounds. Although designed to help people with OA lose weight, AF#8 is equally effective for people with gout. If you have gout and are severely overweight, or you have heart or kidney disease, diabetes, leukemia, psoriasis or any other disease or disorder sometimes associated with gout, your weight-loss program should be monitored by a physician.

Step 2. Get the animal fat and protein and the purines and xanthines out of your diet. Purines in foods form the uric acid which causes gout. Xanthines, found in coffee, are a precursor of uric acid.

Each of the following foods contains 150 to 1000 mg of purines per 3.5-ounce serving. You should permanently eliminate all of them from your diet: alcohol, anchovies, asparagus, beer and wine, bouillon, caviar, clams, coffee, consomme, duck, fish roe, goose, gravies, herring, kidneys, liver, mackerel, meat extracts, meat soup, mincemeat, mushrooms, mussels, organ meats including brains, heart, sweetbreads or tongue, oysters, paté de foie gras, pork and most other rich or fatty meats, sardines, scrabble, shrimp and most seafood, smoked fish or meats, squab, sugar and yeast.

Certainly these are not everyday foods. But they are commonly consumed by those who eat a rich diet. By contrast, most fruits and vegetables, tea, milk and dairy products, eggs, nuts and seeds contain negligible amounts of purines. However, some nutritionists advise people with gout to limit dried peas and beans to one serving per day.

To rid your diet of all rich and fatty foods, read, adopt and practice AF#9: Fewer Pounds Spell Pain-free Joints and AF#10: The One Diet That Does It All.

Step 3. Eliminate alcohol and beer. Alcohol in any form increases uric acid production and inhibits the ability of the kidneys to filter out uric acid. The simplest way to phase out alcohol is to cut your intake by one drink per day until your intake equals zero.

To recover from gout naturally, *alcohol must go*. In studies at the University of Pittsburgh School of Medicine during the 1980s, gout sufferers who ate a meal of rich food experienced only a moderate increase in uric acid levels. But when they consumed whisky and wine with the meal, their uric acid levels soared.

Step 4. Start a daily exercise program that includes both aerobic and strength-training exercise. To get started, read the introductory section of Chapter 6. Then read, adopt and practice AF#5: The Amazing Benefits of Rhythmic Exercise and AF#7: Let Your Muscles Ease the Agony of Arthritis.

A combination of both aerobic and strength-building exercise is essential for weight loss to occur. Work out with strength-building equipment one day and aerobically the next. For as long as you continue to exercise 6 days each week, gout should never be a problem again.

Step 5. Increase your fluid intake so that you are drinking 8 glasses per day. People with gout need more fluid to help uric acid crystals dissolve, to assist in digesting carbohydrate foods, to prevent kidney stones from forming and to minimize the risk of dehydration which can trigger a flare-up of gout symptoms in some people. Among the best fluid sources are plain water, tea (herbal, black or green) or a sports drink.

Step 6. Replace vitamins that are frequently depleted by gout. People with gout are often deficient in vitamins B, C and E. Nutritionists familiar with gout often recommend taking a full-spectrum supplement containing all B-complex vitamins, especially folic acid. For vitamin C, a 250-mg tablet each morning and evening should be more than adequate. And a daily supplement containing 200 to 400 I.U. of natural vitamin E should provide antioxidant protection.

Follow the manufacturer's recommended dosage on each bottle. More may be better when it comes to eating fruits and vegetables, but taking megadoses of any vitamin, especially B or C, could hinder rather than help your recovery from gout. (For more about nutrient needs see AF#14.)

Step 7. An optional folk remedy worth trying is eating half a pound of red or black cherries each day. Fresh cherries are preferred, but canned or frozen usually work well. Some people report good results with cherry juice concentrate or even with extracts sold in health food stores. Many people with gout keep a can of pie cherries in the refrigerator and eat 2 ounces of cherries 4 times a day. Other people mix cherries with other fresh fruits and top them with plain non-fat yogurt to form a delicious fruit cocktail. Usually you must eat the cherries for several weeks before gout symptoms begin to disappear.

Cherries are rich in flavonoids, a nutrient with a powerful ability to lower uric acid levels by alkalyzing the blood. Blueberry, hawthorne and watercress are also rich in flavonoids, and reports show that these foods have also reduced the pain and symptoms of gout. All these are healthy foods that grow on plants, and the more of them you eat, the less room there is for foods of animal origin which contain fat and purines.

Eating cherries or other flavonoid-rich foods works best when followed in conjunction with the other steps in this program. But these foods do help offset the causes of gout. And eating them regularly can't do anything but good.

Follow these steps while you continue to take your antigout medication. As your health improves, your doctor can gradually phase out your medication. Ninety percent of people who adopt and stay with this program for life are able to completely stop taking antigout drugs. About half the remainder are able to reduce their medication by 50 percent.

ARTHRITIS FIGHTER #14: Speed Up Your Recovery
with These Nutritional Heavyweights

No single vitamin or mineral, nor any combination, is
likely to cure arthritis. But numerous studies have shown
that people with arthritis are often deficient in nutrients essential to the integrity of the bone and cartilage in their
joints and to the health of their immune systems. A deficiency of these nutrients can hamper and retard recovery
from OA, RA or gout.

Add together the nutritional depletion caused by emotional
stress and the stress of pain, the chemical action of drugs,
poor absorption of nutrients due to age, nutritional deficiencies
caused by RA itself and the nutritionally deficient Standard
American Diet, and you have some idea of the widespread
nutritional depletion found in most people with arthritis.

Many drugs used to treat arthritis deplete the body of key
vitamins and minerals, especially NSAIDs and immunosuppressive drugs. Anyone taking arthritis medication who also
eats few vegetables and fruits, and who experiences emotional stress, may show signs of suppressed immunity. To
maintain optimal immunocompetence requires a very adequate supply of most vitamins and minerals. The stress
caused by pain alone consumes large amounts of vitamin C.
And with advancing age, poor assimilation and malabsorp-
tion are increasingly common.

Most People with Arthritis Are Nutritionally Deficient

Scores of studies have clearly demonstrated that literally
millions of men and women with arthritis fail to get the
RDA (Recommended Daily Allowance) of most nutrients.
To make matters worse, the RDA listed for each vitamin

and mineral is often the bare minimum needed to sustain life and to prevent diseases like scurvy or pellagra.

For example, a 1995 study at HNRC found that adults need more vitamin D than the current RDA of 200 I.U. To prevent bone loss (often associated with arthritis), researchers concluded that we need at least 400 I.U. per day and possibly as much as 800 I.U. Another study made at England's Salisbury General Hospital in 1985 revealed that at least one-fourth of all people with RA showed evidence of severe malnutrition. Despite eating a so-called well-balanced diet, many of the participants were underweight and had low blood levels of key nutrients such as folic acid and zinc. Researchers concluded that their deficiencies were due to a combination of the RA disease itself and the drugs used to treat it.

While megadoses of vitamins and minerals are not the answer, many individuals may need more vitamins and minerals than the current RDA. Unless you eat at least 16 servings of fruits, vegetables, whole grains and legumes each day, you may well be deficient in vitamins and minerals that could help you to recover from arthritis. For more about the benefits of a plant-based diet, see AF#10: The One Diet That Does It All. No supplement can supply the bonanza of antioxidants, fiber and phytomins—as well as vitamins and minerals—that exist in foods that grow on plants.

If you choose to continue eating the Standard American Diet, which is woefully deficient in vitamins and minerals, most nutritionists recommend taking a multiple vitamin/mineral supplement each day. Nowadays, as growing evidence shows that current RDAs do not meet the nutritional needs of most Americans, more and more nutritionists are recommending that a multi supplement contains 200 percent of the RDA for most vitamins and minerals.

While many supermarket chains and discount houses offer

quality multis at significant savings, none is able to provide *all* the nutrients that most people require. Minerals such as calcium and magnesium, and vitamins C and E, are too bulky to compress into any multi. It's best to purchase these nutrients separately.

FILL IN THE NUTRITIONAL GAPS IN YOUR DIET

Here is a brief review of those nutrients most likely to be deficient in people with arthritis.

- *Vitamin B-complex:* Because they are depleted by stress, the B-complex vitamins are often low in people with arthritis. Since B-vitamins function more effectively when the entire B-complex is taken together, I do not recommend buying individual B vitamins. Any good B-complex supplement should contain at least 400 mcg of folic acid.

  Some people claim to have relieved the pain and symptoms of OA by taking large amounts of the B-vitamin niacinamide. But the amounts required could cause nausea or liver damage. In these quantities, niacinamide becomes a drug rather than a vitamin and should be taken only under medical supervision. Similar claims have been made that vitamin B6, pyridoxene, relieves carpal tunnel syndrome. The dosage required is 100 mg which, though 5 times the RDA, is commonly found in B-complex supplements. If you decide to try it, take it as part of a full B-complex supplement.

- *Vitamin C:* Vitamin C, or ascorbic acid, is essential for the health of bones, cartilage, muscles and blood vessels in joints. Studies show that both inflammation and ar-

222

thritis medications deplete the body's stores of vitamin C. Such a deficiency may be responsible for the easy bruising which afflicts many people with RA. While the overall progress of RA isn't likely to be changed by taking vitamin C, an adequate intake of ascorbic acid is essential, especially during flare-ups.

Researchers in a British study recently concluded that 500 mg or more of vitamin C daily significantly reduced skin bruising common in people with RA, while it also boosted their immune system. Skin bruising was inhibited still more when bioflavinoids were taken together with the vitamin C. Bioflavinoid supplements are available in health food stores, or they can be obtained by eating the pith of citrus fruits together with the rest of the fruit.

Another 8-year study of 640 people with and without OA of the knee at Boston University found that participants who consumed the most vitamin C had barely one-third the cartilage damage of those who ate the least vitamin C. Those with the most disease progression consumed less than 120 mg per day, equivalent to the amount of vitamin C in two oranges. The study's author, Tim McAlindon, M.D., reportedly suspects that by acting as an antioxidant, vitamin C neutralizes the free radicals that are responsible for actually damaging the cartilage in OA. Study results were published in a supplement to *Arthritis & Rheumatism* (September 1995).

Anyone taking NSAIDs, especially aspirin, may require 1,000 mg per day. A fairly high intake of vitamin C can be obtained by eating foods such as citrus, kiwi and other fruits such as strawberries and such vegetables as asparagus, broccoli, Brussels sprouts, cabbage, cauliflower, peppers and sweet potatoes. Millions of people with arthritis eat few, if any, fruits or vegetables and suffer from a serious deficiency of vitamin C.

- *Vitamin D:* The ravages of RA often lead to osteoporosis or loss of density in bones adjacent to an afflicted joint. Some drugs heighten this effect, especially in women. Bone loss can be prevented by including sufficient calcium in the diet. But vitamin D is required to metabolize the calcium.

  Vitamin D is found in milk (but not in all dairy products) and in fatty fish like herring, mackerel, salmon or sardines. You can also mobilize vitamin D by sunbathing for about 20 minutes 3 times a week. However, due to the weakened ozone layer, sunbathing could lead to skin cancer, and sunblock or sunscreen block vitamin D synthesis from solar rays.

  Instead, most doctors recommend taking a vitamin D supplement of 400 I.U. However, the new study from HNRC (cited earlier) suggests that Asian or fair-skinned women with slender builds could use up to 800 I.U. daily. In fact, just about everyone with arthritis could probably use a vitamin D supplement.

- *Vitamin E:* Because it sops up free radicals that damage cartilage in arthritic joints, vitamin E is an important arthritis-fighting nutrient. When used together with other antioxidants, studies have shown that vitamin E has helped relieve the pain of both OA and RA.

  In 1982, the British Arthritic Association conducted a 90-day study of 100 of its members, all of whom had RA, to see if daily supplementation with a variety of antioxidants used together would relieve their pain. The supplements included 45 I.U. of vitamin E, 1,500 I.U. of vitamin A, 90 mg of vitamin C and 100 mcg of selenium. Sixty-four percent of participants reported considerable improvement in pain levels—usually their pain had subsided, though it continued to linger. Those who continued taking the antioxidants after the 90-day period reported further improvement.

Shortly afterwards, a British health magazine conducted another 90-day study of 500 readers with RA. Participants again took the same antioxidants. Results showed that 276 reported an improvement in overall health and 136 experienced a lessening in arthritis pain.

In another study of 29 people with OA made in Israel in 1991, participants took 200 to 400 I.U. of vitamin E each day. Two months later, approximately half reported marked relief from pain.

Most study authors have found that a combination of vitamin E with other antioxidants is more effective than vitamin E alone, perhaps because vitamin E serves as a catalyst to enable other nutrients to function as antioxidants. Unless free radicals are neutralized by vitamin E and other antioxidants, they will continue to damage the cartilage and synovial fluid in joints, leading to loss of lubrication and subsequent inflammation.

The more antioxidants we consume in our diet, the less pain and destruction we're likely to suffer from any form of arthritis. And vitamin E is certainly one of the most powerful and effective antioxidants.

Because it occurs only in foods high in fat, it is almost impossible to consume sufficient vitamin E in the diet without also eating a dangerously high level of fat. The solution, of course, is to take a daily vitamin E supplement containing 200 to 400 I.U. Other antioxidants, which work together with vitamin E, are found in broccoli, celery, dark-green leafy vegetables, mushrooms, yellow-orange fruits and vegetables, wheat germ, whole grains and canned salmon and tuna.

- *Calcium:* Sooner or later, most men and women with arthritis develop osteoporosis or loss of density in bones adjacent to arthritic joints. Asian women and slender, fair-skinned Caucasian women are especially prone to osteoporosis. Bone loss can be prevented by (1) exercising the entire body, including arthritic joints if possible, with a combination of aerobic and strength-building exercises (see AF#5 and AF#7) and (2) consuming 1,000 to 1,500 mg of calcium together with magnesium (see next nutrient) in the diet each day and 400 I.U. of vitamin D. Vigorous exercise is an essential step in preventing osteoporosis.

  The best dietary sources of calcium include dark-green, leafy vegetables, nonfat dairy products—especially plain nonfat yogurt—sesame seeds, tofu and the bones of canned sardines or salmon.

  Painful bone spurs, especially in the heel, may also be associated with various forms of arthritis. Usually, spurs are due to a deficiency rather than a surplus of calcium. Anyone with calcium deposits needs to maintain an adequate intake of dietary calcium and not reduce intake in the belief that the spur will disappear.

- *Magnesium:* The mineral magnesium is vital to the integrity of bone and muscle in joints and also for maintaining a healthy balance in the immune system. The Standard American Diet supplies barely 40 percent of the magnesium requirements of anyone with arthritis, and a magnesium deficiency can cause muscle spasm, a painful condition often associated with arthritis. A daily supplement of 250 mg should protect you against a deficiency. Single combined calcium-magnesium supplements are available.

Although a deficiency of selenium or zinc, or both, is common in people who are under stress or taking medications, these essential minerals are usually included in most multivitamin/mineral supplements.

Let Food and Nutrition Turn On Your Inner Healing Powers

While researching this book I heard, read or was told about a score of different nutrients that various people claimed had helped their arthritis. Vitamin E alone was said to relieve RA. Glucosamine sulfate was recommended for its ability to speed up cartilage repair. One person claimed that the amino acid phenylalanine relieved the pain of OA. All required long-term use in amounts so high that most doctors I talked with advised they be taken only under medical supervision.

Even then, do they really work?

Few have actually been tested in studies controlled for the placebo effect and most reports are anecdotal. Overall, about 30 percent of the people who took these nutrients reported some benefit. This is almost identical with results expected from the placebo effect.

By comparison, the diet, foods and nutrients in our Arthritis Fighters are backed by solid research and studies. I'm not suggesting that you can eat away arthritis or gout. But making dietary changes requires that you act. And as you may recall from Arthritis Fighter #1, when you have full faith and belief in an active therapy, it can turn on the full force of your inner healing power. And that may be enough to put your arthritis into remission.

CHAPTER EIGHT

The Psychological Approach: How to Tap into the Arthritis-Relieving Powers of Your Mind

The most important medical discovery of modern times is that almost every degenerative disease or disorder is a byproduct of unresolved emotional stress.

No disease is more closely linked with stress than rheumatoid arthritis. In fact, RA is often nothing more than the fallout from repressed anger, hostility and resentment. In turn, stress creates an imbalance in the immune system. Pain clinic records describe a number of cases in which women

228

with RA experienced a remission within days of learning how to defuse the stress in their lives.

The basic underlying cause of their arthritis was holding outdated and inappropriate negative beliefs. When we perceive life through a filter of these destructive beliefs, the mind sends self-defeating messages to the immune system that distort its function and trigger RA.

OA and gout are also strongly linked to stress.

True Healing Begins in the Mind

This chapter describes a series of mental action-steps designed to reduce or even to eliminate much of the stress that may be causing arthritis.

Stress reduction works in one of two ways:

1. Coping methods, such as relaxation training or biofeedback, help you let go of stress by learning to relax both body and mind. Coping with stress is quick, easy and successful, but like a tranquilizer, it works only for a day or so at a time. After that, you must repeat the relaxation procedure all over again.

2. Transformational methods prevent stress from occurring in the future. By allowing you to let go of negative beliefs that aren't working and by replacing them with positive beliefs that enhance health and well-being, techniques such as belief reprogramming can almost completely liberate us from stress.

Neither coping with nor eliminating stress can heal the physical damage already caused by arthritis, but they can very definitely retard or even stop further damage. They are also powerful pain relievers. And in an encouraging number of cases, they have caused a complete and lasting remission of RA.

And laughter therapy—the most powerful and successful stress-relieving technique of all—works on both the coping and transformational levels as it knocks out the deep-seated negative beliefs that are the real cause of arthritic disease.

Like all other Arthritis Fighters, stress-management techniques work best when used in a holistic combination with one or more Arthritis Fighters that function on the physical and nutritional levels.

Almost everyone can safely use the psychological action-steps in this chapter. But if you have any emotional problems or emotional instability, if you hallucinate or are schizophrenic, psychotic or prone to hysteria or if you have any other mental or psychological dysfunctions, you should have your doctor's permission before using any of the techniques in this chapter.

Since we often "get" what we visualize or tell ourselves, I strongly suggest that you avoid making any kind of imagery that pictures something detrimental to the eyes, eardrums, joints, muscles or any other organ in the body. It's fine to visualize yourself with improved sight, hearing or health, but never visualize your eyes removed from your head and do not picture a knife or nail being driven into your eyes, ears, heart, brain, arteries or any other fragile organ.

ARTHRITIS FIGHTER #15: The Funnybone Factor: Laugh away Arthritis

---

Since the late Norman Cousins laughed himself back to health after developing a life-threatening autoimmune disease in the 1970s, scientists have been researching the therapeutic benefits of laughter. After measuring laughter's effects on blood pressure, oxygen levels and pulse rate, William Fry, M.D., professor of psychiatry at Stanford University School of Medicine, found that laughter can be as beneficial as exercise and a low-fat diet combined. Although laughter can be performed on a couch, Professor Fry found that laughing exercises muscles all over the body, improves circulation and heart action, oxygenates every cell, stimulates the brain, suppresses stress hormones and enhances immunity.

In another study, Kathleen Dillon, Ph.D. and associates reported in the *International Journal of Psychiatry* (15:13–17, 1985–6) that 10 students viewed a humorous film, then an emotionally neutral videotape. Viewing the humorous film boosted levels of salivary IgA antibodies that defend the body against viral infections, while viewing the tape produced zero results. The authors concluded that people who make humor part of their lives may experience a permanent enhancement of the immune system.

Later studies demonstrated that the act of smiling and laughing induce deep relaxation throughout the body-mind. Tension flows away from taut muscles in the face, diaphragm and abdomen, leaving them deeply relaxed.

Laughing is a whole-person therapy. It reduces immunosuppressors like epinephrine and cortisol and boosts production of endorphins which kill pain and restore balance to the immune system. Laughter is also a powerful analgesic. Ten minutes of deep belly laughs can provide 2 hours of freedom from pain.

Gelotology, as laughter therapy is known, is also the one best way to turn on our inner healing-regeneration system. Laughter therapy, in fact, is the best and fastest way to put RA into complete remission.

The reason is that you can't laugh and feel happy and, at the same time, be stressed out. Because it does exactly the opposite, laughter is the surest way to beat RA.

EIGHT WAYS TO LAUGH YOUR ARTHRITIS AWAY

Practice the following eight techniques and laugh away your arthritis.

1. *Give Yourself a Natural High.* Start off each day with a positive outlook by exercising briskly each morning before breakfast at a pace sufficiently vigorous to release pain-killing endorphin molecules in your brain. This aerobic exercise gives you the equivalent of a runner's high that elevates your mood for the rest of the day. So exercise briskly every day. See AF#1, Step 6: Turn on Your Brain's Feel-Good Mechanism.

2. *Make a Laughter List.* Exactly what turns us on and makes us laugh is something we must each discover for ourselves. Slapstick comedy sends some people into paroxysms of laughter, while others are turned on by more complex sitcoms. Whatever it is that provides you with a good hearty laugh, you need to write down and make a source list of laughter and fun. Then go back over the list, view the video or play the recording or whatever it was, and laugh all over again. That way, you can quickly have yourself laughing whenever you feel a downer approaching.

3. *How to Feel Like Laughing.* You'll feel much more like laughing and having fun if you stop watching violent TV shows and disturbing TV news and give yourself good mes-

sages instead. Phrase each message as an affirmation, such as "I forgive everyone, everything and every circumstance unconditionally, totally and right now." Then experience the relief as the weight of one or more grudges slides from your shoulders.

Or tell yourself, "I choose to enjoy every moment of every day regardless of where I am, what I'm doing, whom I'm with or how I'm feeling." Repeat each affirmation 3 or 4 times several times each day (for details, see AF#18).

4. *Say Yes to Life*. And laugh at all of life's hurdles and inconsistencies. For instance, the next time you're stuck in a long line waiting at the bank or supermarket, visualize the clerk with a tortoiseshell on his or her back. Visualize the man ahead of you growing a beard and see the woman in front of you draped in cobwebs. To make it even more ridiculous, imagine the manager bringing out mattresses and blankets and serving meals and setting up portable toilets as he apologizes for the long time you must wait. When we lighten up and laugh at life's problems, they don't seem so big any more.

5. *Watch Funny Shows*. Go to funny plays and movies and watch slapstick videos or TV comedies that really make you laugh. You need deep belly laughs to turn on your inner healing powers, not just mild amusement. That's why old-time movies like "Candid Camera" or films featuring Buster Keaton, Laurel and Hardy and the Three Stooges are so beneficial. More recent shows featuring the late British comedian Bennie Hill are also hilarious. So are the modern Dorf videos featuring Tim Conway. And there are doubtless many others.

6. *The Zen Morning Laugh*. One of many benefits I discovered while studying Zen is the ability to go through all the physical motions of laughing without having anything

really funny to laugh at. Try it yourself. Sit down and begin to laugh. In a few seconds, you'll feel so good that everything will seem funny and you'll just continue laughing and laughing and feeling better all the time.

7. *Rediscover Your Inner Child.* It's easy to recapture your childlike sense of awe and wonder and your ability to enjoy unexpected things on the spur of the moment without advance planning. Set aside a totally unplanned and unstructured period each day in which you can create, explore, invent and discover. In the process, you'll liberate the joyful, free-spirited child within you.

Throughout this period, drop your mask of adult dignity and let go of all the roles you are playing. Psychologists report that kids laugh 400 times a day, while adults average only 15 laughs a day. So stop taking yourself too seriously. For half an hour each day, forget you're an adult and play at anything you enjoy as if you were young again.

8. *Laugh Yourself Well.* I'll never forget the evening I spent in a class that taught us how to laugh away stress. Right off, we each grabbed a hat and stick and acted like vaudeville hoofers as we danced and cavorted to lively polka music. Then we made faces in a mirror, tossed a ball, tried our hand at juggling and just danced and clapped and jumped around.

It took only minutes to let go and pretend we were kids again. We felt so freed up we could laugh at ourselves and act and look as silly as we wished. That evening was the best antidote to stress I've ever experienced. And the instructor wound up by telling us that many psychologists believe that we reach the peak of self-esteem when we can joke about ourselves and find humor in our own mistakes.

All you need is a room to yourself with a mirror on the wall and some polka music, and you could duplicate this whole routine without anyone seeing you. It's the best stress buster I've ever encountered. The very best thing you can do for your arthritis is to laugh, play, relax and have fun.

Join a volleyball game, fly a kite, model with clay, play with children or a dog. Do something entirely new and different. Join a class in folk or square dancing, country western or rock 'n' roll. Try tubing down a river or go sledding or skiing. Cultivate a youthful curiosity for anything new, exciting and unplanned. And before you know it, you may find yourself wondering what happened to your arthritis.

ARTHRITIS FIGHTER #16: Relaxation Training: Nature's Antidote to Pain and Tension

---

If you've read Chapter 3 ("Stress: A Shapeless Destroyer of Body and Mind") you will already know how the mind turns on the fight-or-flight response whenever it perceives a threat or emergency. Within a second, the entire body-mind is adrenalized. Every muscle is tensed for action. Arteries constrict in our extremities, causing hands and feet to become clammy and cold, while the entire torso becomes so tense that the lungs can no longer move freely and respiration becomes shallow and rapid.

Meanwhile, the brain is jolted into the beta state, an active, hyperalert condition in which the brainwave frequency shoots up to 14 or more cycles per second. It's in this range that arthritis can become exquisitely painful and rheumatoid arthritis flare-ups are frequently triggered.

Each of these factors intensifies muscle tension, anxiety and sensitivity to pain. For example, most people can feel

235

intense pain only when their brainwave frequency is in the beta range of 14 cycles per second or more.

The relaxation response is the exact opposite of the fight-or-flight response. As adrenalin fades away, muscles relax, our extremities feel comfortable and warm and the brain drifts into the reverie-like alpha state of 7 to 14 cycles per second, a range in which intense pain cannot usually be experienced. The mind becomes clear, calm and free of all negative thoughts and feelings, while the respiration slows from 15 to 22 shallow breaths per minute to 6 or 8 deep, slow breaths.

Defuse Pain and Stress with Relaxation

We can turn on the Relaxation Response by using a simple technique called "relaxation training." When we do, we minimize tension and all the other discomforts of stress. We also diminish our sensitivity to any type of stress-related pain, and almost all arthritis pain is stress-related. Pain clinic records show that at least half of all arthritis patients who learn relaxation training are able to reduce or eliminate their pain medication.

In other words, relaxation training lets you transform the pain-provoking fight-or-flight response into its exact opposite, the calming, soothing relaxation response. It works by allowing you to intervene in, and gain control, over a series of involuntary functions of the body that most doctors believe can be accessed only by drugs.

Working at the Menninger Clinic and other medical centers, researchers in behavioral medicine have discovered that when body muscles are tense, the mind becomes anxious and disturbed and its sensitivity to pain is dramatically increased. Yet when body muscles are relaxed, the mind also becomes calm and relaxed and our feeling of pain is much less severe. Likewise, when the mind is calm and relaxed, body muscles also become relaxed, and we feel much less pain.

Relaxation training exemplifies the basic concept of behavioral medicine, which is that we can change the way we feel by changing the way we act. Practice relaxation training and within minutes you can transform stress and tension into calm and relaxation while your arthritis symptoms and pain become much less severe.

Almost Anyone Can Learn to Use Relaxation Training

Before you begin, you must know two things. First, you must be able to recognize muscular tension. And, second, you must know how to use abdominal breathing.

After that, the methods described below take you, step by step, into the deepest level of relaxation that it is possible to reach without drugs. While it takes a few minutes to learn each step, once you know the steps you will find you can attain deep relaxation in less and less time. By following our step-by-step process, in just a couple of weeks you should be able to achieve deep and total relaxation in just 2.5 minutes.

But first, a brief caution: If you have any form of chronic disease, such as hypertension, heart disease or osteoporosis—or if your arthritis is severe enough to be adversely affected by muscle tensing—I recommend you consult your doctor before tensing your muscles as described below.

How to Identify Muscular Tension

Millions of people with arthritis live in such a continual state of muscle tension that they have forgotten what relaxation feels like. During a study at the Menninger Institute

237

in 1986, authors Joseph Sargent and Patricia Selback learned that many of the participants were unaware of how it felt to be truly relaxed. It was only after undergoing a full session of relaxation training that these patients could identify the difference between tension and relaxation.

Before you can use relaxation training, it's essential to recognize how each of these states feels.

Here's how to do it. Lie comfortably on your back on a bed, couch or carpeted floor with a low pillow supporting your head. Keep both your arms and legs straight but relaxed. Your hands should be a few inches from your sides and your feet a few inches apart.

Step 1. Tense and relax your arms. Raise your right arm about 8 inches off the floor, clench your fist and tense your entire lower arm from fist to elbow. Squeeze and tense your muscles and fist as tightly as possible and maintain the tension.

Focus your awareness on the dull ache of any muscle tension in your right arm as you continue to hold it tensed. Hold the tension for only 6 seconds. Then release it and gently lower your arm. Notice how pleasant and comfortable your hand and arm feel as they experience immediate relaxation.

Without stopping, repeat the same routine with your left arm and fist. As you tense your left arm, compare how it feels with your now-relaxed right arm. Keep your left arm and fist tensed for just 6 seconds. Then release and gently lower your arm.

Never again should you have difficulty recognizing the steady ache of muscular tension and the delicious feeling of relaxation.

Step 2. Recognize tension in your face and jaw. Now that you know how tension feels, mentally scan your face, jaw and eyes, looking for areas of tension. Almost all of us can identify the dull ache of tension around the eyes and at the hinge of the jaw. Many people with arthritis experience chronic tension in the face, jaw, eyes and forehead.

To tell if you are relaxed, ask yourself these questions. Do I feel peaceful and content? Is my mind clear and calm? Has all tension gone? Do I feel rested and relaxed? A "yes" answer to each usually indicates you are in the relaxation response.

Melt Away Tension with Abdominal Breathing

Whenever we're anxious or stressed, we take rapid, short and shallow breaths. That's because stress triggers tension in the muscles. And as muscles in the neck, chest and abdomen are contracted by tension, they prevent our lungs from moving freely. Actually, this is a mechanism of the fight-or-flight response and its immediate effect is to make us feel pain much more intensely than when we're relaxed.

Decades ago, yoga instructors discovered that we can swiftly defuse stress and pain by breathing in exactly the opposite way. Whenever we inhale through the nose and take deep, slow belly breaths, our lungs send messages to the brain that turn on the relaxation response.

Taking deep, slow belly breaths is also known as abdominal breathing. Usually, it takes only a few minutes of abdominal breathing to achieve a significant reduction in muscle tension and a noticeable decrease in any pain we are feeling.

Anyone who studies yoga swiftly discovers that abdominal breathing revitalizes the entire body-mind. For this reason, I suggest that you attempt to slow your respiration to 4 to 8 breaths per minute whenever you practice relaxation training.

239

To practice abdominal breathing, sit on an upright chair with your legs uncrossed and your hands in your lap. Alternately, you can sit cross-legged on the floor. Inhale through your nose if you can. While practicing abdominal breathing, count silently once per second.

Step 1. Inhale deeply to the count of 4, filling the abdomen and bottom of the lungs first, then the middle chest and finally the upper chest. As you inhale, place one hand on your abdomen and the other on your upper chest. If breathing correctly, you will feel your abdomen expand during the first second of inhalation and your upper chest expand during the fourth second.

Step 2. Hold your breath to the count of 4.

Step 3. Exhale. Take at least 4 seconds, or longer if you like, to exhale. As you exhale, empty your upper chest first and your abdomen last. Smile as you exhale and visualize tension flowing out of your body.

Assuming that the full inhale-exhale cycle takes 12 seconds, this totals only 5 breaths per minute. This is much slower than the 15 to 22 short, shallow breaths many of us take when we're anxious or stressed.

As you breathe, focus your awareness on the breath. "Watch" the breath as it flows in and out through your nostrils.

Not everyone is able to slow her or his respiration to 5 breaths per minute. So stop if that feels unnatural. Just breathe as slowly and as deeply as you can in a way that feels comfortable. Return to normal breathing immediately if you feel nauseous or dizzy.

Yet if you inhale for 2 seconds, hold 2 seconds and exhale

for 2 seconds, you are still breathing only 10 times a minute. That's usually slow enough to calm your mind and keep you in the relaxation response.

FOUR SIMPLE STEPS TO DEEP RELAXATION

To make it easy to learn, pain clinics often teach relaxation training in 4 simple stages.

1. Tensing and relaxing each muscle in the body one at a time.
2. Deepening your relaxation.
3. Relieving arthritis pain with a simple visualization.
4. Taming stress and pain with biofeedback.

In practice, you simply flow on without interruption from stage 1 to stages 2, 3 and 4. If for some reason you are unable to tense your muscles, omit stage 1 and use only stages 2, 3 and 4.

STAGE 1. TENSING AND RELAXING EACH MUSCLE IN THE BODY ONE AT A TIME

By tensing each muscle group in the body as tightly as possible for 6 seconds and then releasing, you burn the stored-up energy that is keeping your muscles tense and contracted.

Step 1. Go to the bathroom, wipe your hands and face with a damp washcloth and empty your bladder. Then go to a quiet room where you will not be disturbed and unplug the phone.

Step 2. Lie on your back on a comfortable bed, sofa or carpeted floor with a low pillow under your head. Keep your arms and legs extended, with your hands a few inches from your sides and your feet a few inches apart. Begin to breathe deeply and slowly.

Step 3. Frown as hard as you can and look upward. Hold 6 seconds and relax.

Step 4. Press your tongue against the roof of your mouth, screw up and tense all of your face, and close your eyes and tense your eye muscles. Tense all these areas tightly for 6 seconds, then relax.

Step 5. Press the back of your head down against the pillow and arch your neck and shoulders off the bed or floor. Hold 6 seconds, then relax. Next, roll your neck loosely from side to side several times.

Step 6. Tense your neck and shoulder muscles as tightly as you can. Hold 6 seconds and relax.

Step 7. Tense your chest muscles as tightly as you can. Hold 6 seconds, then relax.

Step 8. Raise your right arm about 6 inches off the bed or floor. Keep your arm straight. Clench your fist tightly. Then tense your muscles tightly all the way from your shoulder down your bicep and forearm to your fist. Hold 6 seconds, then relax. Gently lower your arm.

Repeat with your left arm.

Step 9. Raise your right foot 6 inches off the bed or floor. Tightly tense your entire leg from buttocks to toes. Curl your toes tightly if you can. Hold 6 seconds, and relax. Then gently lower your leg.

Repeat with your left leg.

Step 10. Tightly tense both buttocks simultaneously. Hold 6 seconds and relax.

Step 11. Tightly tense your back and abdomen muscles. Hold 6 seconds and relax.

Step 12. Take 6 slow, deep breaths. At each inhalation, visualize a soft, green healing light flowing in through the soles of your feet, moving on up your legs and spreading to every part of your body. At each exhalation, visualize any lingering tension flowing out of your body and leaving through the soles of your feet.

Step 13. Roll your eyes slowly from side to side several times, then up and down, and relax.

By now, you should be in a state of deep muscle relaxation. Continue on without pause to stage 2.

STAGE 2. DEEPENING YOUR RELAXATION

Now that you've released all physical tension, Stage 2 uses suggestions and visualization to deepen your relaxation. Repeat the suggested phrases silently to yourself while you create a mental picture of the limb or muscle deeply relaxed. Don't try to force or hurry anything. Just keep repeating the suggestions and "seeing" the visualizations in your mind's eye. Then just let it happen. If another thought or daydream intrudes, slide it aside and return to your imagery.

Step 1. Place your awareness on the soles of your feet while you silently repeat to yourself, "My feet feel loose, limp and relaxed. Waves of relaxation are flowing into my feet. My feet are warm and deeply relaxed. Relaxation is flowing into my feet and legs. My feet and legs are loose, limp and relaxed. Waves of relaxation are flowing into my thighs. My thighs feel loose and limp and relaxed. My legs, feet and thighs are filled with comfort, warmth and pleasure. "

You need not repeat the exact words, but use essentially the same message. Focus your awareness on the area you

243

are relaxing. Visualize it as loose, limp and relaxed. Some people prefer to visualize their legs or thighs filled with cotton and the area as limp and relaxed as a piece of tired old rope. Continue to repeat the suggestions and imagery until your muscles or limbs feel completely relaxed.

At first, you will find it easier to relax one leg at a time. Should you still detect any area of tension, mentally relax it before you continue.

Step 2. Next, focus your awareness on your buttocks and repeat to yourself, "Waves of relaxation are flowing into my buttocks. My buttocks feel limp, loose and relaxed. My buttocks are filled with comfort, warmth and pleasure."

Repeat the same suggestions and visualizations for your back muscles, abdomen, chest and shoulders and for each arm.

Step 3. Focus your awareness on your neck and face as you tell yourself, "My scalp is limp and relaxed. My forehead feels smooth and relaxed. My eyes are quiet and relaxed. My face is soft and relaxed. My tongue and mouth are limp and relaxed. My jaw is slack. My neck is loose and relaxed. I feel comfort, warmth and pleasure in every part of my face and neck."

The face and neck are doubly important since tension appears here before it appears anywhere else in the body. By relaxing your eyes and jaw, you can often induce relaxation in other body parts. So doublecheck your eyes and jaw for any hint of lingering tension.

Step 4. Experience the soothing comfort of relaxation around your eyes and "feel" it flowing into the eyes themselves. Feel waves of comfort, warmth and pleasure radiating through your scalp and forehead, down to your ears, into the back of your head and neck and on down into your cheeks, nose, mouth, tongue and jaw.

Your entire body should now feel soft, limp, loose and relaxed. Enjoy the feeling of comfort, warmth, pleasure and well-being.

When you are ready, continue without pause to stage 3.

STAGE 3. RELIEVING ARTHRITIS PAIN WITH A SIMPLE VISUALIZATION

You can now deepen your relaxation by using a simple imagery technique that will relax your mind and reduce your sensation of pain.

Step 1. Visualize yourself in a beautiful garden filled with flowering trees and shrubs. You are standing at the top of a wide marble stairway. The stairs lead down to a deep, clear spring. So transparent is the water that you can see every detail on the white sandy bottom 50 feet below.

The stairway has 12 steps. Slowly descend the stairs. As you reach the first step, begin to silently count backwards from 12. For instance, at the second step, say "eleven." Count backwards as you descend the remaining steps. As you count zero, you should be standing beside the spring.

Step 2. Now toss a shiny new dime into the clear water. Watch the coin dart, turn, glide and flash as it descends slowly through the water. In your imagination, stay about 2 feet from the dime and watch it twist, roll and dart as it slides down and down, deeper and deeper into the silence of the spring. After about a minute, the dime comes to rest on the white sandy bottom.

Step 3. You are now at the deepest part of the spring, completely insulated from stress, noise, problems, deadlines or pressures of any kind. Here, far from freeways and telephones, all is completely calm, still, tranquil and relaxed.

Say to yourself, "My mind and body are deeply relaxed. I feel only peace, love and joy. I am completely at ease and in harmony with nature. There is nothing I need or want. And there is nothing I have to do. I feel completely content and I am filled with comfort, warmth and pleasure."

Although your mind feels deeply relaxed, you should be wide awake and aware of everything that is going on. If any thoughts of the past or future intrude on your mind, let them slide off. Keep your awareness focused on the here and now and continue to enjoy the present moment.

You can continue to rest and enjoy your deeply relaxed state or you can flow on without pause into biofeedback, therapeutic imagery or belief restructuring. Or you can return to normal consciousness.

To Return to Normal Consciousness

When you choose, open your eyes and move them up and down and from side to side. Open and close your jaw. Raise and lower your eyebrows. Then give a wide grin. Raise and lower your head and roll it from side to side. Curl and uncurl your fingers and toes. Then move each muscle, one by one. Sit up slowly and turn from side to side. Finally, stand up slowly.

Try to avoid any sudden movement while returning to normal consciousness and for a few minutes afterward. This should help the benefits of deep relaxation last for several hours. For relief from arthritis pain, deep relaxation should be practiced twice daily, before breakfast and again in late afternoon. As a prophylactic to prevent pain from occurring, one session a day is usually sufficient. You can also use deep relaxation to help get to sleep or go back to sleep at night.

A Faster Way to Reach Deep Relaxation

Relaxation can't be hurried or rushed. To make it work, you must be able to identify stress and use abdominal breathing. You must also begin by using all 3 stages of relaxation training. Each time you use it, your body "learns" to relax in less and less time. Most fit people are soon able to tense every muscle in the body simultaneously. This shortcut reduces the time needed for muscle tensing to under 15 seconds. Then by combining visualization with a series of 8 slow abdominal breaths, you can reach a deep level of relaxation in just 2.5 minutes.

It's done like this.

Step 1. Lie on your back on a bed, couch or carpeted floor with your arms and legs extended. Begin abdominal breathing. Keep your legs straight and together. Then raise both feet about 8 inches off the bed or floor. Without pausing, raise your trunk until your shoulders are also about 8 inches off the bed or floor. Stretch your arms out in front of you, parallel to the floor.

Step 2. Take a deep breath and begin to exhale. As you breathe out, tense every muscle in your body simultaneously. Curl your toes and tense your feet, calves, thighs and buttocks. Tense your shoulders, back, chest and abdominal muscles. Clench your fists and tense your arms and hands as tightly as you can. Tense your entire face, mouth, tongue, eyes, forehead and neck muscles.

Hold all your muscles at maximum tension for 6 seconds. Then let go and lower your entire body gently back to the floor.

If you find steps 1 and 2 rather difficult at first, try tensing your muscles while standing. Simply stand erect, or lean forward with your knees bent and your hands on your knees. Then tense every muscle in your body for a brief 6 seconds, and release. As you let go, lie down gently on the rug, couch or bed.

Whether you tense while standing or lying down, you will need to practice this method several times. It's best learned in easy stages. For example, begin by tensing first one leg, then the other, and finally both legs together. Then, one by one, add the arms, shoulders, chest, back, abdomen, buttocks and the neck and face.

When you can do that, begin to tense and release all the muscles above your waist simultaneously. Next, tense and release all the muscles below your waist simultaneously. With a little practice, you should soon be able to tense every muscle in your body at the same time, hold for 6 seconds, and release.

You'll find muscle tensing much easier if you exert yourself only while exhaling.

Step 3. All your muscles should now be relaxed while you continue to breathe slowly and deeply, using abdominal breathing. With your first inhalation, visualize a soft, green healing light entering your body through the soles of your feet and flowing swiftly on up through your legs and torso to your neck and face. As you briefly hold your breath, "feel" your neck and face becoming limp, loose and relaxed. As you exhale, picture all the tension flowing out of your face and leaving your body through the soles of your feet.

Step 4. With each successive abdominal breath, use the same technique to mentally relax each of the following areas:

1. Relax your neck and face.
2. Relax your left arm.
3. Relax your right arm.
4. Relax your shoulders, back, chest and abdominal muscles.
5. Relax your buttocks.
6. Relax your left leg and foot.
7. Relax your right leg and foot.

With each breath, place your awareness on the area you are relaxing and visualize the soft, green healing light flowing to that area. Take a final deep breath as you silently tell yourself, "I am warm, comfortable, happy, calm and completely relaxed."

Based on this program, it should take only 7 deep breaths to mentally relax your entire body.

At 15 seconds per breath for 8 breaths, plus 15 seconds for muscle tensing, the entire relaxation process can easily be done in 2.5 minutes.

You can now continue without pause to stage 4, biofeedback.

STAGE 4. TAMING STRESS AND PAIN WITH BIOFEEDBACK

Doctors who work in pain clinics often regard biofeedback as the ultimate technique for coping with stress or alleviating the pain of arthritis. In tests at Laval University in Quebec, biofeedback reduced pain in patients with arthritis in their hands by 50 percent. Those with RA also decreased their sedimentation rate and reduced their need for medication.

Biofeedback consists of learning to dilate the arteries in your hands through the use of verbal suggestions and mental images.

First, you use all 3 stages of relaxation training to become deeply relaxed. Then, by silently repeating verbal suggestions while you make mental pictures of your hands as warm and relaxed, you saturate both your brain's left and right hemispheres with a single message. That message is to warm your hands. Since your mental pictures and your verbal suggestions are unconditionally accepted by the brain, they are swiftly transformed into physical action.

In a few minutes, arteries and capillaries in your hands begin to relax and dilate, allowing more blood to flow into your hands. This literally makes your hands heavier and warmer. After a few practice sessions, the effect begins to generalize and arteries all over your body begin to relax and dilate. The immediate effect is you let go of tension.

Tense people usually have cold, clammy hands. That's because their fight-or-flight response is constricting arteries that supply blood to the hands. As blood flow is reduced, the hands become clammy and cold. By creating exactly the opposite effect, biofeedback turns off the fight-or-flight response and restores the relaxation response. In the process it also warms the hands.

A New Dimension in Arthritis Relief

Biofeedback is widely used by pain clinics because of its proven ability to reduce every kind of stress-related pain. Most pain clinics have a biofeedback lab equipped with state-of-the-art monitoring devices. If you can obtain professional biofeedback training of this caliber at affordable cost, you should certainly get it. Otherwise, you can obtain surprisingly good results using the do-it-yourself method described below.

To practice biofeedback, make sure the room temperature is at least 72° F and your hands are moderately warm. If your hands are cold, immerse them in a basin of warm water for 2 minutes to restore circulation; then towel them dry.

To begin biofeedback, you must first use relaxation training to become deeply relaxed. You can use either the full 3-stage method or the faster way. In either case, you should be lying on a bed, couch or carpeted floor thinking of nothing in particular but just enjoying your state of complete relaxation. Then, without pause, flow into the following steps.

Step 1. In your mind's eye, create a pleasant, restful scene in which you see yourself lying in the warm sun on a tropical beach. In your imagination, experience all the sensory feelings, sights, sounds and smells that are part of this scene.

Picture the white sails of several fishing boats on the aquamarine sea. "See" flecks of white cloud floating in the wide blue sky. "Feel" the caressing breeze and "hear" it murmuring through the palm trees. Experience the warm, heavy feeling of relaxation as it spreads throughout your body.

Feel the texture of the sun-warmed sand beneath your hands and feel its warmth flowing into your fingers and palms.

Step 2. Focus your awareness on your fingers and hands and repeat these phrases silently.

"My hands and fingers feel heavy and warm."

"Warmth is flowing into my hands."

"My hands feel quite warm."

"My hands and fingers feel warm and relaxed."

"My fingers are tingling with warmth."

"My palms and fingers are glowing with warmth."

"My hands and fingers are heavy and warm."

Keep repeating these, or similar phrases, while you continue

251

to visualize waves of warmth, heaviness and relaxation flowing into your hands.

Step 3. In just a few minutes, the fingers of one or both hands should begin to tingle, a reliable indicator of artery dilation. As soon as you detect a tingling in one hand, mentally magnify that feeling. Then in your imagination, "transfer" that feeling to your other hand.

As your fingers start to tingle, tell yourself, "My hands are heavy and tingling with warmth. The tingling in my hands is quite strong. I feel calm, relaxed and warm all over."

If you have any difficulty, focus on warming only one hand or only one finger on one hand. If you can warm a single finger, it proves you have good biofeedback abilities.

Once you are able to warm both hands, you can go on to include your forearms in your biofeedback training. Later, you can use the same kind of imagery and suggestion to warm your feet and legs as well as your hands and arms.

Affordable Aids to Improve Biofeedback

You can check your hand temperature by touching your hand to your face before beginning the biofeedback session and again at the end. Your hand should feel noticeably warmer. However, more accurate feedback devices are available that measure microscopic changes in the perspiration and temperature levels of your hands. These hand-held devices provide actual feedback to help monitor your progress during relaxation.

One such device is a hand-held galvanic skin response (GSR) monitor that measures the extent of perspiration on your skin by producing a tone that becomes lower in pitch as your tension level diminishes. Another is an electronic digital readout thermometer that displays the temperature of a hand or foot in tenths of a degree.

Both of these devices provide immediate feedback that enables you to detect subtle movements in hand temperature and relaxation level far smaller than is otherwise possible. Neither device is essential, but they can help you learn to relax and warm your hands in appreciably less time.

You can also listen to a prerecorded audio cassette tape instead of repeating your own silent verbal suggestions. Recorded by a professional hypnotist, these tapes take you swiftly into deep relaxation and then into hand-warming. You can also record your own tape. One advantage of listening to a tape is that you cannot hurry, or try to speed up, the relaxation process.

Tapes and GSR or skin temperature monitors are often advertised in health, biofeedback, headache and hypnotist magazines or perhaps on the Internet. Or you may locate them through suppliers such as Self Care (see Appendix).

Let Nature Help You Tune Out Stress

Between relaxation training sessions, you can help stay relaxed by getting and staying in touch with nature. Stress is heightened by losing contact with nature and by living indoors, driving cars and watching TV. Being enclosed by walls and windows frequently increases anxiety and stress.

Instead, spend as much time outdoors as you can. Walk among trees and on grass, barefooted if you like. Feel the wind and the rain on your face. Look at inspiring panoramas and views. Listen to the wind rustling leaves, the surf, a stream or falling rain. Watch the stars by night and the clouds by day. Experience the stillness and the subtle changes of color at sunrise and sunset. All are soothing

253

sounds and sights that help tune out the modern world and its harsh and stressful realities.

When you're ready, you can use deep relaxation as a springboard to therapeutic imagery, described in AF#17.

ARTHRITIS FIGHTER #17: How to Heal Your Arthritis with Therapeutic Imagery

---

At first, medication had helped Joan control the excruciating surges of pain in her shoulder caused by RA flare-ups. But as time went on, most pain-killing drugs relieved Joan's pain for only a few days. Then their effectiveness steadily diminished. Finally, nothing seemed to work.

In desperation, Joan sought help at a local pain clinic.

"I wake up hurting so badly I want to scream," she told the doctor.

"What does the pain feel like?" he asked.

"Like a red hot dagger plunged into my shoulder," Joan replied without hesitation.

"What would take your pain away?" the doctor asked.

Joan thought a moment.

"A bag of ice cubes cold enough to make my shoulder turn blue," she said.

Joan was instructed to lie down on a couch. She was told to keep her eyes closed and take several deep breaths and relax.

"Now visualize a red-hot dagger plunged into your shoulder," the doctor told her.

In her mind's eye, Joan pictured a dagger, its blade glowing red with heat, stuck deep into her arthritis-stricken shoulder.

"Now imagine the dagger being withdrawn very slowly,

254

just half an inch at a time," the doctor instructed. "When the dagger is completely withdrawn, mentally picture a frigid icebag draped across your painful shoulder."

As Joan carried out the visualization, the doctor spoke again.

"In your imagination, 'feel' and 'see' the ice numb your shoulder until your skin turns blue," he told her.

Joan was then instructed to silently repeat the following verbal suggestion: "The pain and inflammation in my shoulder are gone. As the icebag numbs my shoulder, I no longer feel any pain at all. I feel perfectly comfortable and at ease."

It took only a few minutes for Joan to complete the visualization. As she finished, she realized that, for the first time in weeks, the pain in her shoulder was noticeably less severe.

"The pain relief won't last forever," the doctor told her, "but whenever your flare-ups return, you can use this same therapy again."

The Awesome Healing Power of Therapeutic Imagery

Joan had just completed her first session of therapeutic imagery, also known as guided imagery or visualization. So awesome is its healing power that many experts at pain clinics consider visualization the most powerful pain-relieving tool in the entire arsenal of natural therapies.

Therapeutic imagery has proven so successful that it is often used in hospitals to help patients recover faster from operations and lessen the need for pain-killing drugs after surgery. But it also helps people with arthritis in a variety of ways.

Visualization is often used by sports psychologists to train athletes for the Olympics and other world-class events. Millions of Americans use visualization programs such as "inner

255

golf," "inner tennis" or "inner swimming," all based on making mental pictures of successful sports techniques and then reinforcing them with silent verbal suggestions.

For instance, you can perfect a new swimming stroke just as effectively by visualizing yourself using it as by actually practicing the stroke in a pool. As you mentally rehearse a sports routine in your mind, you activate the same areas of the brain, and you build the same neural pathways, that you would use if you actually did it.

Before I drove a rental car through England, I used visualization for several evenings to rehearse driving on the left, overtaking on the right and negotiating traffic circles with half a dozen exits.

Normalize Your Immunity with Visualization

Therapeutic imagery for arthritis relief works in much the same way. You make clear mental pictures of your desired goal or you "see" yourself performing an Arthritis Fighter technique. Then you reinforce your imagery with silent but strongly positive verbal phrases and suggestions. By communicating in symbol language with the right brain and in verbal language with the left, you create an inner dialog that bypasses the conscious mind and saturates the subconscious with your message.

Since the subconscious uncritically accepts all images and suggestions that we make, it communicates our wishes to every gland, nerve, muscle and organ in the body. Powerful inner forces then begin to work subliminally to transform our goals into reality.

Now a respected psychological tool, therapeutic imagery can be used in a variety of ways to help overcome arthritis. Since the immune system responds swiftly to mental images, it is hardly surprising to find that some people have learned to control at least one aspect of their immune systems. (As you may recall, an imbalance in the immune system is usually responsible for setting off RA.)

For example, a series of studies by Karen Olnes and colleagues, documented in the *International Journal of Neuroscience* (63:221–234, 1993), demonstrated that by practicing visualization, a person could learn to control at least one aspect of the immune system. Participants in the study were taught to induce deep relaxation, then visualize an image of white blood cells called "neutrophils." These cells defend the body against bacteria or fungus infections and they also play a key role in provoking autoimmune diseases such as RA.

To reduce the possibility of autoimmunity, participants were instructed to immobilize their neutrophils by visualizing them as sticky. One participant visualized her neutrophils as ping-pong balls covered with honey so they stuck to everything they touched. When blood samples were tested afterward, results showed that people who practiced the relaxation-visualization therapy successfully were able to selectively increase the stickiness of their neutrophils.

A similar study at UCLA School of Medicine demonstrated that after practicing relaxation-visualization techniques, participants with malignant melanoma showed significant increases in the number and activity of natural killer cells that are part of the cancer-slaying immune system.

Therapeutic imagery is even more successful when we use it to change behaviors that affect the competence of our immunity. For example, exercise clearly helps strengthen and restore balance to the immune system. But if you lack the motivation to take a brisk daily walk, you can empower yourself to begin a walking program by visualizing yourself enjoying a walk each day. Or by visualizing yourself carrying out any of the physical or nutritional Arthritis Fighters in this book, you can swiftly motivate yourself to begin doing them.

Call it self-hypnosis if you like, but the brain will automatically carry out whatever instructions we give it while we're relaxed and using therapeutic imagery. That's because what we "see" and what we "say" to ourselves is what we get.

Visualization works best when we are deeply relaxed. In fact, pain specialists often refer to it as relaxation-visualization. Thus your first step is to become deeply relaxed, exactly as described in AF#16. After practicing AF#16 for a couple of weeks, you should easily become deeply relaxed in 2.5 minutes. In fact, many people are able to relax their entire body-mind in only 1 minute.

By relaxing the body, you also relax the mind and you enter a state of focused attention. Instead of wandering from thought to thought, your mind becomes completely absorbed in your imagery and suggestions. All other thoughts are excluded.

Once relaxed, you simply begin making mental pictures of whatever it is you wish to achieve while you reinforce these images with silent verbal suggestions. In some cases, imagery alone may accomplish your goal and verbal suggestions may not be required.

However you employ therapeutic imagery, use images and suggestions that portray your goal as already accomplished. To motivate yourself to walk 3 brisk miles each day, visualize yourself as already walking 3 miles daily and use suggestions that reinforce it.

To relieve arthritis pain, use images and suggestions that show your pain as already gone. Do this, even though your pain still exists. Phrase and visualize everything you wish to do as though it were already an accomplished fact.

Isn't this denial, you may ask? The answer is "no." Visualizing yourself free of pain is not the same as denying you have it. Denial doesn't do any good. In fact, denial may cause you to put off seeing a doctor or fail to take proper care of yourself. Instead, therapeutic imagery merely supplies your body-mind with a blueprint to guide it to total wellness.

Make Vivid, Graphic Images

For best results, all images should be as clear, realistic and detailed as possible. Choose scenes and symbols that bring alive your feeling of being free of arthritis.

One of the most powerful visualizations is to picture yourself in perfect health with a trim, athletic build and striding along a beach without a single ache or pain anywhere in your body. As you "see" yourself walking along the beach, use your imagination to "experience" sensory impressions that reinforce the emotional content of your images.

For example, mentally experience how good it feels to be lean, light, flexible and free of pain. As you "see" yourself striding along the beach, "feel" the grains of sand under your feet. In your imagination, "hear" the screech of gulls as they wheel overhead and "smell" the tang of salt in the air.

Although I don't have arthritis, I often visualize myself working out with weights. As I lift a barbell at least 10 pounds heavier than any I have lifted in real life, I "hear" the metallic clink of the barbell and weights. And when I visualize myself swimming faster than I ever have in reality, I "hear" the hiss of water surging past my ear.

If you work out on strength-training machines in a gym rather than with free weights, you can still "experience" similar sounds and feelings. Involving all the senses in your imagery makes your mental pictures more alive, and it makes your visualization far stronger and more effective.

See Yourself As Already Healed

Your silent verbal suggestions should be strongly positive. Use the present tense and speak as though you had already achieved your goal.

For example, phrase all suggestions as though your arthritis had already disappeared. Telling yourself "My arthritis will disappear tomorrow" sounds weak and vague compared with the powerful suggestions used by Joan in the case history described earlier. Speaking in the present, Joan told herself: "The pain and inflammation in my shoulder is gone. As the icebag numbs my shoulder I no longer feel any pain at all. I feel perfectly comfortable and at ease."

Do as Joan did, and use only active, positive words. Telling yourself "My entire body is relaxed at all times" is far more effective than "I will never feel tense again."

Avoid beginning a suggestion with "I would like to . . ." or "I don't . . ." or "I won't . . ." It's far more effective to tell yourself "I am walking 3 brisk miles each day" than "I would like to walk 3 miles each day."

Choose phrases that express feelings, and endeavor to express those feelings as you continue to make images. Telling yourself that "I am happy and delighted to be walking 35 minutes each day" lets you "experience" these same strongly positive feelings as you continue to visualize yourself walking each day.

Likewise, a phrase such as "Becoming a nonsmoker has made me really proud of myself" empowers this suggestion with strongly positive feelings.

Repeat each suggestion at least 4 times during each imagery session and say it slowly, silently and clearly. Repeat each phrase with anticipation and enthusiasm and avoid a reticent or hesitant style.

How to End a Visualization Session

As you end your visualization session, experience gratitude that your inner healing powers have overcome arthritis. Really *feel* grateful and thankful as you repeat phrases such as "I feel comfort, pleasure, health and happiness in all my joints and muscles. I am happy, delighted and thankful to be free of arthritis pain."

Lastly, congratulate yourself for having taken a completely active step in your own recovery. Tell yourself: "I feel terrific, optimistic, cheerful and filled with energy. As I think, feel, say, imagine and believe, so I become. Every day in every way I am getting better and better."

These are extremely important steps in making the visualization process work and invoking your inner healing-regeneration powers. So always end each visualization session by expressing deep and genuine thankfulness for your recovery from arthritis, even though in real life you may still have arthritis pain and symptoms.

Most people can make graphic images that are sufficiently vivid and clear that they work well in visualization. If you wonder whether your imagery powers are good enough, try this brief experiment.

Sit down, relax and close your eyes. First, visualize a snow-capped mountain peak. Next, visualize a red setter dog. Finally, visualize a yellow tulip. Hold each image for a short while.

If you were able to make reasonably strong, vivid images

of each of these subjects, and were able to hold them in your mind for at least a brief while, you probably have excellent visualization abilities. But even if your imagery is less than perfect, you may still use visualization successfully. What really counts is the effort you put into making the images and suggestions and the extent to which you sense and experience their content.

What to Do If You Can't Visualize

Endless hours of passive, mind-dulling TV watching does impair our creativeness and our ability to make images. So if you find visualization really difficult, try this. Simply sit down with pen and paper and describe your imagery in writing.

The mere act of writing automatically produces vivid mental pictures and strong images. So write out your verbal suggestions as well. Also draw a sketch of yourself walking, stretching, bicycling or eating a green vegetable salad or whatever else your goal may be.

Even people who can visualize well have improved their results by describing their arthritis-recovery steps in writing instead of just viewing them as pictures in their mind.

To return to normal consciousness, take a deep breath. As you exhale, count back slowly from 5 to 1. Beginning with your eyes and face, slowly move each muscle and limb in turn. Then sit up and remind yourself that, as your images take hold and begin to work, you must be prepared to do whatever it takes to reach your goals.

Visualization can be tremendously helpful in relieving arthritis. It provides powerful motivation and it helps you rehearse every kind of physical or nutritional action-step. But it can't replace worn cartilage, increase the range of motion of your joints or provide your body with disease-fighting nutrients. Where exercise and nutrition are concerned, you must be prepared to do in real life what it actually takes to relieve your arthritis.

VISUALIZATION 1: IMAGERY FOR CONTROLLING ARTHRITIS PAIN

Similar to that used in the case history of Joan, described earlier, this powerful imagery technique can be employed to relieve arthritis pain almost anywhere in the body.

Step 1. Once deeply relaxed, ask yourself four standard questions. The answer should be intuitive, meaning the first thing that crosses your mind. These are the questions, with some typical intuitive responses.

Question 1: What does my pain feel like?
Intuitive answer: An electric drill boring into my spine.
Question 2: What color is the pain?
Intuitive answer: An ugly, pulsating purple.
Question 3: What would relieve my pain?
Intuitive answer: Switching off the power, then pulling the drill out and applying an icebag.
Question 4: What color would my back be then?
Intuitive answer: A cool, soothing shade of blue.
Step 2. For a brief few seconds, visualize the drill boring into your spine and "feel" the pain at the spot where it is most intense. Mentally picture the painful area surrounding the drill and "see" your flesh as ugly, pulsating and purple.
Step 3. Visualize a hand turning off the switch to the drill and "hear" a loud click as the power is turned off. Next, a quarter of an inch at a time, visualize the drill slowly being withdrawn from your spine. Simultaneously, repeat silent verbal phrases like "As the drill is withdrawn, I feel less and less pain. The drill is no longer boring into my back and I feel better already."

Step 4. Once the drill is completely withdrawn, "see" and "feel" an icebag draped over the painful area. A cool, soothing light blue color then spreads into your flesh, displacing the pulsating purple color. Reinforce these images by repeating such phrases as "The ice is numbing my back. I no longer feel any pain. The pulsating purple color has gone. My back is now a soothing, pain-free blue. The blue color has driven away the pain. I am completely free of pain and I feel terrific."

While using this visualization, your intuition may portray the source of your pain as an axe, sword, spear, saw, knife, hammer, red-hot iron, crushing weight or knotted muscle. You then visualize that object at the location of your pain, with the flesh surrounding it suffused by the color of your pain. Visualize the object of your pain being slowly withdrawn, or otherwise removed, from your flesh. Finally, picture your pain-relief object soothing the pain while the pain color fades away and is replaced by the pain-relief color.

For severe pain, consider practicing this visualization 3 times each day. Most people, however, find that practicing once a day is enough to reduce most arthritis pain by one-third and, after a week, by one-half. By then, pain relief usually lasts several hours. The more you practice, the greater the relief and the less time it takes you to relax and do the imagery.

VISUALIZATION 2: TO RESTORE BALANCE TO A DYSFUNCTIONAL IMMUNE SYSTEM

You can reduce risk of developing an autoimmune disease such as RA by using the neutrophil visualization described earlier under "Normalize Your Immunity with Visualization." But therapeutic imagery is even more successful when we use it to boost factors such as our self-image that directly influences the balance and competence of our immune system.

Some specialists in behavioral medicine believe that restoring the balance and competence of your immune system is the surest way to achieve a remission from rheumatoid arthritis. The one best way to accomplish that is by sending the body-mind a strong message about your health goals and how you want to look and feel.

Step 1. Recall how you looked and felt at the healthiest period of your life. Recall how easily and painlessly you moved, how great you felt about yourself and how satisfied, content and fulfilled you were.

Step 2. Visualize yourself in this state of high-level wellness, striding or jogging along a beach, confident that your immune system can swiftly repel any disease or infection. "See" yourself as lean, fit, suntanned and athletic. Involve all your senses as you picture yourself in this super-healthy state.

"Feel" the sand crunch under your bare feet, "see" the gentle surf cream over your toes, "hear" the screech of gulls circling overhead and "smell" the tang of salt in the air. You're feeling superb, without a trace of stiffness or pain, and every joint in your body has full freedom of movement. You're completely healed; you can't be sick. Picture yourself laughing, feeling youthful, relaxed and having fun.

If you prefer, visualize your own version of a healthy scene. You might see yourself playing tennis in Hawaii, cross-country skiing in Colorado, mountain biking in Utah or doing whatever else your arthritis may have prevented.

Step 3. It's important to conclude this particular visualization by expressing gratitude for your liberation from arthritis and for having been healed. Be certain to feel and express gratitude, even if in reality your arthritis still exists.

Feel deeply grateful as you say: "I feel pleasure, health, happiness and comfort all over my body. I am happy and grateful to be free of arthritis pain and symptoms."

Wind up by congratulating yourself for having played an active role in your own recovery. Tell yourself: "I feel terrific, cheerful and optimistic, and I am completely free from arthritis pain. As I think, feel, image, say and believe, so I become. Every day in every way I'm getting better and better."

VISUALIZATION 3: FIND OUT EXACTLY WHAT IS CAUSING YOUR RHEUMATOID ARTHRITIS

"I felt like curling up and dying" was how Betty described one of her frequent flare-ups of rheumatoid arthritis. When her doctors were unable to explain why these flare-ups occurred, Betty consulted a behavioral psychologist.

The psychologist told Betty that her best chance of finding out was to consult her "inner guide." Betty was instructed to enter deep relaxation, then to visualize a blank bedroom wall that contained only a closet door. When the closet door swung open, Betty's inner guide would be revealed behind it. The guide might be a person, a religious figure, a rabbit, wise owl, crow or other animal.

The psychologist explained that our inner guide is actually a symbol of our own deepest self. Our inner self can access the deepest levels of the body-mind including our memory banks and belief systems. Our guide can take us on a mental journey of self-discovery deep into the interior of our subconscious minds or into the vast array of memories stored in our memory banks. A dialog with our inner guide may reveal penetrating insights into the source of arthritis pain and provide helpful guidance on how we can heal it.

The psychologist also told Betty that whenever she asked her inner guide a question, the first thing to enter her mind afterwards would be the answer.

When the closet door swung open, Betty's inner guide turned out to be a wise old man with a long white beard. When Betty greeted him in silent verbal language, she learned that his name was Porbananda. Betty asked Porbananda what caused her rheumatoid arthritis and flare-ups and what she might do to obtain a remission.

Porbananda replied by pointing to a rowboat tied to the bank of a small lake. Betty and Porbananda sat down in the rowboat and Porbananda rowed out into the lake. Then he stood up and dived overboard.

Almost a minute went by before Porbananda's head broke the surface. He reached out of the water and handed a round white object to Betty.

"This is the cause of your rheumatoid arthritis," Porbananda said, "and also the cure."

Then Porbananda slid back into the water, and this time he did not reappear.

When Betty examined the round white object, she recognized that it was a large wall clock. But the clock had no hands and the plain white face was completely blank.

Puzzled, Betty wondered how this could explain her RA flare-ups and pain. Suddenly, she understood. Her problem was hurry sickness. She lived by the clock and she was always under pressure and running late.

Her fast-paced lifestyle was causing such excessive stress that it triggered her immune system to begin attacking the cartilage in her joints.

267

As Betty realized that Porbananda had provided her with the guidance she sought, she experienced tremendous relief. Starting the next morning, she scheduled a more relaxed workday, with less pressure and fewer deadlines and she set aside a period for exercise each day.

Gradually, over the following weeks, Betty's RA began to subside and eventually she achieved total remission. Using similar imagery, Betty was able to renew contact with Porbananda. And she used her inner guide's advice to achieve even higher levels of healing and wellness.

This story, in which I was personally involved, tells it all. If you prefer, you may meet your inner guide by visualizing a small lawn covered by an opaque white cloud. As a puff of wind blows the cloud away, your inner guide will be revealed.

If you choose to duplicate Betty's imagery, you may also meet your inner guide and discover the cause of your RA (or almost any other pain or disorder). Several other people I know who used this technique had the causes of their RA revealed by their inner guides. Their causes ranged from an unhealthy relationship to feeling resentful and working at a stressful job. When the cause was eliminated, each person soon achieved a permanent remission from RA. Caution: This technique is not intended as a substitute for a medical diagnosis.

VISUALIZATION 4: RELIEVE OSTEOARTHRITIS BY LOSING WEIGHT

Visualizing the steps you must take to lose weight can be a great help in motivating you to actually do so. Imagine yourself performing any of our Arthritis Fighters, and if you don't soon begin to do it in real life, you may start to feel slightly uncomfortable.

Step 1. Visualize yourself working out on a strength-training machine in a gym, preferably one that involves doing abdominal crunch-ups. "Feel" your abdominal muscles work and "hear" the clink of the crunch machine each time you do a crunch-up.

Simultaneously, tell yourself: " My muscles are bigger and stronger then ever. Working out becomes easier every day and I enjoy it more and more. As my muscles grow in size, they burn up more fat and they increase my metabolism."

Step 2. Visualize yourself striding briskly along a beach. Use the same imagery and suggestions as in step 2 of Visualization 2.

Step 3. Picture yourself enjoying a large green salad packed with shredded carrots, tomatoes, broccoli, cauliflower and other healthful vegetables. The dressing is completely nonfat. Experience the crisp, crunchy texture and the honest flavor of each vegetable as you eat it, and realize that the salad tastes incredibly good.

Tell yourself: "Natural foods taste wonderful. I enjoy food much more when I know it benefits my health and helps me lose weight."

Step 4. Visualize yourself as lean, suntanned, fit, athletic and without a hint of surplus weight. As in step 2 of Visualization 2, involve all your senses as you picture yourself in this superbly healthful state.

Meanwhile, tell yourself: "I am happy and grateful to have reached my ideal weight. My knees are free of arthritis pain. And I feel pleasure, health, happiness and comfort all over my body." Then congratulate yourself for having played an active role in your own recovery.

VISUALIZATION 5: NUMB ARTHRITIS PAIN WITH MENTAL ANESTHESIA

When pain medicine proved almost useless, Jonathan learned to numb the pain of his arthritis flare-ups with mental anesthesia. He did so by using a visualization technique known as "glove anesthesia." His pain relief lasted only 30 minutes at first. But after 2 weeks of practice, it lasted several hours. Eventually, Jonathan found he could produce glove anesthesia without having to use either relaxation or visualization. However, for glove anesthesia to work, the pain must be in a fairly compact area, such as the knee.

Step 1. Imagine yourself seated in a comfortable chair and feeling deeply relaxed. In your imagination, visualize a bucket of steaming hot water at the left side of your chair and a bucket of frigid, ice-cold water at the right side.

Mentally picture yourself immersing your left hand in the bucket of hot water. "See" the water steaming and "feel" your hand tingling with warmth. Tell yourself: "My left hand is heavy and warm. My left hand is tingling with warmth. My left hand feels very warm."

Step 2. As soon as your left hand feels warm, picture yourself removing it from the bucket. Right away, visualize yourself plunging your right hand into the imaginary bucket of ice water. "Feel" the intense, piercing cold and experience immediate numbness, accompanied by total loss of feeling.

Repeat to yourself: "My right hand is numb and cold. My right hand is tingling with frigid cold. My right hand has lost all feeling of pain."

Step 3. Transfer the pain-numbing cold from your right hand to the area of your arthritis pain. Visualize yourself laying your right hand on the painful joint. "Feel" the pain-free numbness flowing from your right hand into the hot, swollen joint. Experience the pain diminishing as the painful area is numbed.

Silently repeat: "I have transferred the pain-numbing cold to my painful area by touching it with my cold hand. Now the joint is numb with cold and free of pain. I have anesthetized the pain with freezing cold and my arthritis pain has disappeared."

Almost everyone who tries this visualization experiences a pain-numbing feeling in the affected joint and pain begins to disappear. Should the numbness fade from your right hand, visualize yourself replacing it in the ice-cold bucket.

At first, you may have to repeat steps 2 and 3 several times. But, eventually, people with RA in the knee, for example, are able to quench their pain by merely taking a few abdominal breaths to relax and then laying their right hand on top of their knee. Then, the reduction of pain usually lasts several hours.

To return to normal consciousness, visualize yourself shaking your cold right hand several times to "shake" out the cold and restore warmth and feeling. (Caution: This entire technique takes place in your imagination while you are lying down; under no circumstance should you use real buckets of either hot or cold water.)

In AF#18 you'll learn how to use an even more powerful type of therapeutic imagery, one that exorcises the stress-provoking beliefs that so often are the root cause of most types of arthritis.

ARTHRITIS FIGHTER #18: Shoot Down Arthritis with Positive Beliefs

Research into the field of psychoneuroimmunology has confirmed that our emotions are the largest single influence on our health. And arthritis is no exception. Every type of arthritis has an emotional component, and in every case, the emotion is negative.

The Root Cause of Rheumatoid Arthritis Lies in Our Beliefs

When we perceive the world through a filter of negative beliefs, we experience negative thoughts. Negative thoughts then trigger negative emotions such as fear, resentment, anger, hostility, guilt, envy, anxiety, frustration or disappointment. Whenever we experience one of these destructive feelings, the mind recognizes it as threatening and sets off all or part of the fight-or-flight response.

Stress hormones then create uncomfortable tension in our muscles while neuropeptide molecules convey messages about how we feel to every cell in our immune system. Immediately, the immune system begins to mimic the way we feel. Negative feelings impair the immune system and distort its functions. Instead of defending the body against cancer and infections, the immune system turns on the body's own cells and begins to attack them. When the immune system targets cartilage in a joint, this abnormality is known as "rheumatoid arthritis."

This chain of cause and effect clearly demonstrates that most cases of RA are caused by stress mechanisms turned on by negative thoughts and emotions that arise from holding negative beliefs.

Not Everyone Who Is Stressed Gets Rheumatoid Arthritis

In most people, stress mechanisms create muscular tension that produces discomfort throughout the body, especially in the stomach. For millions of people, the simplest way to relieve the discomfort of stress is by using food as a tranquilizer. Sweet or fatty foods quickly relieve the discomfort of stress by elevating blood sugar levels.

272

Food may not be a drug, but overeating has adverse side effects of its own. Many people who continually eat to relieve negative feelings—including loneliness, boredom or frustration—eventually become seriously overweight. As the years go by, their excess body weight places an unbearable stress on cartilage in the spine, hips, ankles and knees. As this stress wears away the cartilage, the result is osteoarthritis.

This chain of cause and effect also clearly demonstrates that most cases of OA are caused by stress mechanisms triggered by negative thoughts and emotions that in turn arise from holding negative beliefs.

New Beliefs, New Health

In direct contrast, holding positive beliefs causes us to think positive thoughts that trigger positive emotions such as love, joy and compassion. The brain perceives these feelings as nonthreatening and guides the body-mind into the relaxation response in which arthritis and pain are seldom experienced.

Thus the underlying cause of most cases of arthritis lies in the type of beliefs we hold in our minds. This may be news to the average physician, but thousands of the nation's most prominent neurologists, psychologists, physiatrists, physical therapists, cardiologists, oncologists and even some rheumatologists are acutely aware of it. The reason is that all these health professionals are practitioners of behavioral medicine.

When health professionals of this caliber recognize that stress-provoking negative beliefs are the root cause of diseases like arthritis, their conclusions cannot be ignored. Nowadays, belief reprogramming is widely taught at conferences and workshops on behavioral medicine.

273

Beliefs that involve unforgiveness are considered a prime cause of such destructive emotions as anger and hostility. For this reason, workshops such as "Forgiveness, an essential component in health and healing" or "How beliefs have the power to change your body" are regularly scheduled at workshops and conferences sponsored by organizations like the National Institute for Clinical Application of Behavioral Medicine.

Worn-out Beliefs Can Wreck Your Health

Our beliefs determine how we perceive the events in our lives and whether we see them as hostile and threatening or as friendly and harmless. Depending on our beliefs, the same event can provoke the fight-or-flight response in one person and the relaxation response in another.

For example, due to downsizing, both Smith and Jones were permanently laid off from their jobs. Smith perceived his layoff as a total disaster. He believed his job loss was permanent and he feared he would lose his home, car and furniture.

Jones, by contrast, perceived his unemployment as a heaven-sent opportunity to train for a new career in the computer field.

It wasn't the job loss that was stressful. It was Smith's negative belief system that programmed him to regard his unemployment in a negative way—in a way that triggered his fight-or-flight response and that plunged his entire body-mind into a chronically stressful emergency state.

When Jones perceived the same event through a filter of more positive beliefs, he saw it as nonthreatening and as a welcome opportunity to strike out for a rewarding new career.

Give Yourself an Arthritis-Resistant Personality

Modern life is filled with potential conflicts arising out of money, jobs, relationships or similar life events. Thus it's hardly surprising that people who hold negative beliefs tend to have a much higher incidence of RA, OA and gout as well as cancer, heart disease and other chronic afflictions.

Our beliefs mould our personality and they make us who we are. But the wonderful thing is that if we aren't satisfied with our personality configuration, we can easily change it. If we have a negative personality, prone to stress and arthritis, we can easily transform it into a positive, stress-free personality by reprogramming our beliefs.

Doing so won't rebuild cartilage already damaged by arthritis. But it may well be the best way to achieve a total remission from RA. And it *can* end the stress that causes people to worsen OA by continually overeating.

Unforgiveness Can Wreck Your Health

In our violent and competitive society, millions of people have grown up with the belief that to forgive someone is wimpish. Karen had typically grown up with the belief that she should never forgive an injustice. Karen felt badly cheated when, instead of promoting her to the job for which she was next in line, her boss gave the job to his niece, who was a young college graduate with no work experience.

Whenever Karen thought about how unjustly she had been treated, she would immediately feel tense and uncomfortable. But she saw no reason to forgive her boss and she continued to feel resentful week after week.

275

When Karen woke up one morning, her wrists felt on fire. Her doctor diagnosed it as RA and prescribed a series of pain-killing drugs. Despite this, Karen's RA spread into her shoulders and the pain slowly worsened.

While waiting in her doctor's office one day, Karen read an article in a health magazine about behavioral medicine. The author described how negative emotions like fear and resentment could provoke stress-related diseases such as cancer and RA. Though far from convinced, Karen phoned the 800 number quoted in the article and located a behavioral psychologist in her city.

A week later Karen was seated in the psychologist's office describing her arthritis symptoms. The psychologist didn't seem too interested in the physical symptoms.

Instead, the psychologist asked Karen whom she was mad at.

"My boss, of course," Karen blurted out. "I was treated most unjustly. I'd worked for his company for almost 8 years. I was next in line for promotion to department head. But instead of giving me the job, my boss gave it to his niece, an inexperienced girl fresh out of college. It makes me furious just to think about it. I'll never forgive him. Somebody's going to pay for this."

The psychologist looked straight at Karen.

"Somebody already *is* paying for it," she told Karen. *"You are."*

Karen still had difficulty accepting that it was her resentment and unforgiveness that were responsible for her RA.

"Then forgive your boss," the psychologist said. "I mean *really* forgive him. What have you to lose but your arthritis and all the inappropriate beliefs you've been carrying around in your mind for years? Whether an act is just or unjust depends on how you look at it. Condemning your boss didn't hurt him. You are the one who has suffered. It's your nega-

276

tive beliefs, and the destructive emotions they produce, that are causing your arthritis."

Karen felt angry at this explanation. But something deep inside told her that the psychologist was right.

"I know these beliefs are destroying me," Karen admitted. "Can you help me forgive my boss and get rid of my arthritis?"

In the next hour, Karen learned the basics of relaxation-visualization. The psychologist then taught her a therapeutic imagery technique specifically designed for restructuring beliefs.

It took only two visualization sessions for Karen to completely forgive her boss. As she let go of her resentment, she realized that injustice was merely a fabrication in her mind. An enormous weight seemed to slide from her shoulders. For the first time in months, she felt completely relaxed and free of muscular tension.

In the days that followed, Karen's arthritis pain and inflammation gradually subsided. She did have two more mild flare-ups. But each time the pain was briefer and less intense. The last flare-up occurred 2 years ago and Karen hasn't felt a twinge of pain or inflammation since.

Nowadays, as soon as she experiences any type of conflict or stress, Karen completely forgives the person concerned. She simply witnesses the event without making any judgments and without becoming emotionally involved. By not becoming upset, she is better able to help solve the conflict.

Karen is well aware that her new beliefs and values are not currently embraced by our money-driven culture. But, she feels, not following the mainstream is a small price to pay for staying free of rheumatoid arthritis.

The therapeutic imagery that the psychologist taught her for reprogramming beliefs is described below.

A *Secret Zen Visualization for Reprogramming Beliefs*

To replace a negative belief with a positive belief, imagine yourself in a Zen temple in Japan. "See" yourself sitting cross-legged on the tatami-mat floor. Directly in front of you a flame is burning on a low brass pedestal. "Smell" the perfume of burning incense and "hear" the temple bell and the chanting of monks in the distance.

Step 1. Begin by destroying the negative belief that is causing your stress and arthritis. On your left, see a scroll lying on the floor. Pick it up and unroll it. Written inside in English is the negative belief that is causing your arthritis.

Typically, it might read: "I'll never forgive my brother for what he did to me."

Hold the scroll over the flame and watch it burn. "Smell" the paper burning.

A bare-headed monk wearing a brown robe comes forward. In his hands is a brass bowl. Empty the ashes from the paper into the bowl and the monk withdraws.

Step 2. Install a new positive belief in your mind. To your right, see another scroll lying on the floor. Pick it up and unroll it. The scroll is blank. Using a thick marker pen, write the new belief that will end your arthritis pain and suffering. Your new belief is the first thing that enters your mind. For example, you might write: "I forgive my brother now, completely, unconditionally and always. I also forgive myself for having judged him in the first place."

What your brother did, or how unjust it seemed, is unimportant. You don't have to see or contact him. Simply forgive him. The alternative is to go on suffering.

Read your new belief slowly 3 times as you absorb it and experience it.

Again, the monk comes forward and takes the scroll.

"The new belief is etched in your memory," he tells you, "and it will remain there forever. "

How to Identify Negative Beliefs

Whenever you feel tense or upset, try to recall what you were thinking about just before that occurred. The clues below should help you recognize the type of negative belief that frequently triggers the fight-or-flight response.

- Negative beliefs cause us to feel angry, hostile or resentful about another person or to carry a grudge.
- They cause us to love, accept and approve another person only when that person meets our conditions.
- They are concerned primarily with getting and receiving.
- They cause us to expect a reward for almost everything we do.
- They cause us to compare ourselves with others and to feel dissatisfied and discontent when another person appears to be more successful or to be getting more than we are.
- They cause us to feel insecure, either financially or in our relationships with others.
- They permit us to blame others for things we do and for things that happen to us.
- They cause us to be judgmental of others and to attack, criticize or condemn other people.
- They make us feel resentful or guilty about something we did in the past, or to become worried and anxious about what may happen to us in future.
- They cause us to have strong likes and dislikes, to be rigid and inflexible and to hold strong opinions.

279

Beliefs that match these patterns are usually based on fear. They may have had some validity once, but most have far outlived their usefulness. For as long as we continue to allow them to run our lives, they will continue to provoke stress and a series of diseases ranging from RA or OA to cancer, heart disease and diabetes.

When holding on to a negative, fear-based belief is causing distress, it's obviously time to get rid of it. So surrender its ashes to the Zen monk and replace it with a positive, love-based belief that is its diametrical opposite.

Outdistance Arthritis with These Positive Beliefs

Most positive beliefs are framed as affirmations. To minimize stress and arthritis symptoms, I recommend adopting some or all of the 10 groups of affirmations below. As you read them, you may recognize that you hold an opposite viewpoint or belief. If you feel constantly stressed, or have arthritis, you may well benefit from letting go of the negative belief that is responsible and replacing it with a diametrically different positive affirmation. Use the Zen temple visualization and reprogram only one belief at a time.

1. I relieve my arthritis pain and symptoms as I let go of fear and replace it with unconditional love. I love everyone unconditionally, most especially myself. I accept everyone the way they are without requiring them to change.

2. I recognize that lasting happiness and fulfillment come only from being content and not from things I do, buy, eat or drink. Thus I do and acquire only things that will maintain and deepen my inner peace. I cease craving superficial excitement and stimulation. When I am content and at ease, my body-mind is calm, centered and relaxed. Thus I make choices and decisions only when I am calm and relaxed.

3. I know that absolute security is unobtainable. Yet I always have everything I need to enjoy the present moment. Thus my needs and wants are few. Excluding my occupation, I never expect a reward for my actions. I never seek fame, recognition or praise, and I refuse to do anything to win another person's approval. I also recognize that giving and receiving are the same. Whatever I give away or lose, I will receive back several times over. (Note: This does not apply to gambling, betting, "loaning" money to a financially irresponsible person, including a member of your own family, or giving away money of any amount without careful consideration and thought.)

4. I can only win when everyone wins. Therefore I think in terms of cooperation rather than competition. Instead of competing, I will relax and enjoy every moment of every day regardless of where I am, how I'm feeling, whom I'm with or what I'm doing. To free myself from envy, I avoid comparing myself with others or with their possessions or accomplishments. I am willing to celebrate the good and the successes achieved by others without feeling jealous.

5. I view each seeming problem as a challenge and a fresh opportunity to progress, grow and learn and not as a fight against the clock, another person or a corporation. I accept complete responsibility for who I am, for everything I do and for almost everything that happens to me.

6. I realize that time does not heal wounds unless I actively forgive. Thus I forgive and release anyone I have not forgiven, including myself. I forgive everyone, everything and every circumstance totally and right now. Nor do I expect to be always treated with justice and fairness. I realize that these are qualities that exist in the mind, and I am ready to forgive anyone whom my mind perceives as unfair or unjust.

7. Whether in thought, word or deed, I cease to judge, criticize or condemn another person. I see only the best in

everyone, including, and most especially, myself. I experience a profound oneness with other people and I refuse to see myself as separate or different. Whenever I meet another person, I look for the similarities between us rather than the differences.

8. I have totally ceased to worry about the future. All my fears about the future exist only in my imagination. I am a powerful person and I am completely capable of handling whatever the future may bring. Besides, when it arrives, the future will have become the present. I also totally let go of the past and with it all guilt and resentment.

9. I am always optimistic, hopeful, cheerful and positive. I expect good things to happen to me today, tomorrow and throughout life. I recognize that to exist is bliss, to be here is joy and to be alive is pure happiness. Joy and bliss are my birthright, and I can enjoy them endlessly unless I permit a fear-based belief to influence my thoughts.

10. My birthright is perfect health and freedom from arthritis and other diseases. Perfect health is my normal, natural state. To achieve it I am willing to use my mind and muscles to do whatever it takes to succeed. I am never intimidated by any minor discomfort or inconvenience nor by physical or mental exertion. Above all, I always act as if it is impossible to fail.

Make Yourself Arthritis-Proof

Affirmations like these may seem oddly out of place in a society in which violence and revenge are featured in hundreds of books, movies and TV shows each week. But until 200 years ago, RA was virtually unknown. Today, incidence of all forms of arthritis is increasing faster than in any previous period. And it just may be because of a parallel increase in stress, pressure, crime, isolation and the intolerable pace of life in our modern society.

When you analyze the cause of stress in your life, you will find that most of it is caused by perceiving the world through beliefs that are the very opposite of those in the affirmations just listed.

The choice is yours.

You can choose to embrace the belief and value system of our angry, violent, competitive, aggressive society and go on suffering and popping pills. Or you can choose to make a complete paradigm shift and adopt a positive belief system that gets rid of most of the stress in your life.

To do so, use the Zen temple technique to discover the negative belief that is most responsible for causing your stress. Then, in the same visualization, replace it with an opposite but strongly positive belief. Repeat the visualization once each day for a week. When you feel confident that this belief has been replaced, use the same method to identify your second most destructive belief. Replace that, too, with a diametrically opposite positive belief. Then keep on reprogramming one negative belief each week.

In addition to using the Zen temple imagery, you can repeat the new, positive affirmation to yourself at intervals during the day. For best results, focus on only one affirmation at a time.

What If Your Arthritis Fails to Improve?

Suppose, after trying all the appropriate Arthritis Fighters in this book, your arthritis doesn't improve. If you are among the relatively few arthritis sufferers who cannot be helped by the methods in this book, the worst you have done is outlay the book's modest cover price.

In return, you should have upgraded your lifestyle habits to the point where they cannot fail to improve your overall health. According to the best sources of medical and U.S. government opinion, you should have significantly reduced your risk of ever developing cancer, diabetes, heart disease, hypertension, obesity, osteoporosis, stroke and most other chronic diseases that afflict Americans in their later years.

No one can guarantee that any specific therapy will work for everyone. Your doctor gives no guarantee that his or her medication will ease your pain and leave no side effects.

What I do believe is that this book presents the most complete array of promising nondrug arthritis therapies ever to appear within the pages of a single book. And if you're the average lay reader it should prove to be the most definitive work ever written to help you stop arthritis now.

APPENDIX

The following organizations may be of interest to anyone with arthritis. Addresses and phone numbers were current at press time but may change with the passage of time.

Arthritis Foundation
PO Box 19000, Drawer Al
Atlanta GA 30326
Ph. 800-283-7800

Publishes the bimonthly magazine *Arthritis Today* and a number of helpful and inexpensive books on exercise and other self-care aspects of arthritis. Can direct you to local chapters which provide referrals to doctors, clinics, exercise classes and support groups in your area and to physical and occupational therapists, nurses, social workers and other health professionals.

Self Care
5850 Shellmound St.
Emeryville, CA 94608-1901
Ph. 800-345-3371

Supplies equipment and products for wellness, pain relief and biofeedback and cassette tapes for relaxation and visualization.

Yoga Journal
PO Box 469018
Escondido, CA 92046-9018
Ph. 510-841-9200
   Excellent source for books, tapes and instruction in yoga and yoga exercise equipment.

SELECTED BIBLIOGRAPHY

Adams, John D. *Understanding and Managing Stress: A Workbook in Changing Lifestyles.* Pfieffer, 1980.

Arthritis Foundation, eds. *Understanding Arthritis: What It Is; How It's Treated; How to Cope with It.* Scribner's, 1986.

Baggish, Jeff. *How Your Immune System Works.* Ziff-Davis, 1994.

Barnard, Neal, M.D. *The Power of Your Plate.* Book Publishing, 1990. *Foods That Cause You to Lose Weight.* Magni, 1992.

Barry, Helen. *Imagine Yourself: Using Imagery to Get Well.* Ashley Books, 1990.

Beech, H. R., et al. *A Behavorial Approach to the Management of Stress.* Wiley, 1982.

Benson, Herbert. *The Relaxation Response.* Random House/Value, 1992. *Timeless Healing: The Power and Biology of Belief.* Scribner's, 1996.

Brewer, Earl, and Kathy C. Angel. *The Arthritis Sourcebook: Everything You Need to Know.* Lowell House, 1994.

Brewerton, Derrick. *All about Arthritis: Past, Present and Future.* Harvard University Press, 1992.

Brower, Anne C. *Arthritis in Black and White.* Saunders Press, 1988.

Burns, David, M.D. *The New Mood Therapy*. William Morrow, 1990.

Charlesworth, Edward A., and Ronald G. Nathan. *Stress Management: A Comprehensive Guide to Wellness*. Ballantine, 1985.

Cohen, Darlene. *Arthritis: Stop Suffering, Start Moving*. Walker, 1995.

Cramer, Kathryn D. *Staying on Top When Your World Turns Upside Down*. Viking Penguin, 1991.

Culligan, Matthew J., and Keith Sedlacek. *How to Avoid Stress Before It Kills You*. Random House/Value, 1991.

Decker, John L. *The Reliable Healthcare Companion: Understanding and Managing Arthritis*. Avon, 1987.

Dell Medical Library Staff. *Free Yourself from Chronic Arthritis*. Dell, 1990.

Eliot, Robert S. *A Change of Heart: Converting Your Stresses to Strengths*. Bantam, 1994.

Ellert, Gwen. *The Arthritis Exercise Book: Joint-by-Joint Exercises to Keep You Flexible and Independent*. Contemporary Books, 1990.

Evans, William, M.D., and Irwin Rosenberg, M.D. *Biomarkers: The Ten Keys to Prolonging Vitality*. Simon & Schuster, 1991.

Everly, George S., and Daniel A. Girdano. *The Stress Mess Solution*. Prentice-Hall, 1981.

Fernandez-Madrid, Felix. *Treating Arthritis: Medicine, Myth and Magic*. Plenum Press, 1989.

Ford, Norman D. Titles in Keats Publishing's series *Eighteen Natural Ways to: Beat the Common Cold* (1987), *Beat a Headache* (l990), *Lower Your Cholesterol in Thirty Days* (1992), *Beat Chronic Tiredness* (1993), *Look and Feel Half Your Age* (1996), *Stop Arthritis Now* (1997), *Supercharge Your Immunity* (forthcoming in 1998). Also *Painstoppers*

(1994) and *The Sleep Rx (1994)* published by Prentice-Hall/Reward Books. *The Fifty Healthiest Places to Live and Retire (1991)* published by Ballantine. *Walk to Your Heart's Content (1992)* published by W. W. Norton.

Fries, James F., and Kate Lorig. *The Arthritis Helpbook: A Tested Self-Management Program for Coping with Your Arthritis and Fibromyalgia.* Addison-Wesley, 1995.

Gach, Michael R. *Arthritis Relief at Your Fingertips: A Guide to Easing Aches and Pains Without Drugs.* Warner Books, 1990.

Garrett, Laurie. *The Coming Plague: New Diseases in a World Out of Balance.* Virago Press, 1995.

Gillespie, Peggy R., and Lynn Bechtel. *Less Stress in Thirty Days.* New American Library/Dutton, 1987.

Goodacre, J., and Carson Dick. *Immuno-pathogenetic Mechanisms of Arthritis.* Kluwer Press, 1988.

Gorden, Neil F. *Arthritis: Your Complete Exercise Guide.* (Cooper Clinic Fitness Series). Human Kinetics Press, 1993.

Greenberg, Mark H., and Lucille Frank. *Doctor, Why Do I Hurt So Much? How to Combat Your Arthritis or Arthritis-Like Condition and Start Enjoying an Active Life.* Chronimed Press, 1992.

Hall, H., L. Minnes and K. Olness. "The Psychophysiology of Voluntary Immuno-Modulation." *International Journal of Neuroscience* 69:221-234, 1993.

Hills, Margaret. *Curing Arthritis: More Ways to a Drug-Free Life.* Transaction Publications, 1992.

Janeway, Charles A., Jr., and Paul Travers. *Immunobiology: The Immune System in Health and Disease.* Garland Publishing, 1994.

Kiecolt-Glaser, J. K., et al. "Slowing of Wound Healing by Psychological Stress." *Lancet* 346:1194-96, 1995.

Langer, Ellen J., Ph.D. *Mindfulness.* Addison-Wesley, 1990.

Levine, Norman, M.D. *Skin Healthy.* Taylor, 1995.

McCarty, Daniel. *Arthritis and Allied Conditions: A Textbook of Rheumatology.* Williams & Wilkins, 1992.

McIlwain, Harris H., et al. *Winning with Arthritis.* Wiley, 1991.

McQuade, Walter, and Anne Aikman. *Stress: What It Is. What It Can Do to Your Health. How to Handle It.* New American Library/Dutton, 1993.

Maskowitz, Reed C. *Your Healing Mind.* Avon Books, 1993.

Mehta, Silva, et al. *Yoga: The Iyengar Way.* Knopf, 1990.

Moyer, Ellen. *Arthritis: Questions You Have—Answers You Need.* Peoples' Medical Society, 1993.

Murray, Michael T. *Arthritis: How You Can Benefit from Diet, Vitamins, Minerals, Herbs, Exercise and Other Natural Methods.* Prima Publications, 1994.

Nakayama, T., et al. "Inhibition of the Infectivity of Influenza Virus by Tea Polyphenols." *Antiviral Resources* 21:289-99, 1993.

Newnham, Rex E. *Away with Arthritis.* Vantage Press, 1994.

Nuernberger, Phil. *Freedom from Stress, a Holistic Approach.* Himalayan Publications, 1981.

Phelan, Nancy, and Michael Volin. *Yoga after Forty.* Harper & Row, 1965.

Phillips, Robert H. *Coping with Rheumatoid Arthritis (1988). Coping with Osteoarthritis (1989).* Avery Publications.

Pisetsky, David S., and Susan F. Trien. *The Duke Medical Center Book of Arthritis.* Fawcett, 1995.

Rooney, Theodore, and Patty Rooney. *The Arthritis Handbook.* Ballantine, 1986.

Rothblatt, Henry B., et al. *How to Stop the Pain of Arthritis.* Compact Books, 1985.

Satchidananda, Swami. *Integral Yoga Hatha.* Holt, Rhinehart & Winston, 1970.

Savage, Fred L. *Osteoarthritis*. Station Hill Press, 1989.

Seigman, Martin, Ph.D. *Learned Optimism*. Pocket Books, 1992.

Shen, Harry, and Cheryl Solimini. *Living with Arthritis: Successful Strategies to Help Manage the Pain and Remain Active*. New American Library/Dutton, 1993.

Sinatra, Stephen, M.D. *Heartbreak and Heart Disease*. Keats Publishing, 1996.

Snyder, C. R., Ph.D. *The Psychology of Hope*. Simon & Schuster, 1994.

Sobel, Dava. *Arthritis: What Works*. St. Martins, 1991.

Taylor, Rene. *Yoga: The Art of Living*. Keats Publishing, 1975.

Vishnudevananda, Swami. *The Complete Illustrated Book of Yoga*. Julian Press, 1970.

Williams, Redford, M.D. *The Trusting Heart*. Times Books/Random, 1989. *Anger Kills*. Times Books/Random, 1993.

INDEX

293